Dr. ^fred^ Jung & Trosch
— I do inital programing for ET

Dr. Jones Midland - closest
        ET
— I do initial programing for ET

U of M   Dr. Chou mouent d/o neurologist
         Dr. Patel N-surg

Henry Ford Elen Air ucsf
       Pyskonia N-surgery
       EAIR1@hfhs.org
       313 574-7546 cell

Neurology adjustingDr.Sdiropoulos

Deep Brain Stimulation Management

Deep Brain Stimulation Management

Edited by

William J. Marks, Jr.
University of California, San Francisco

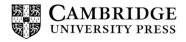

CAMBRIDGE UNIVERSITY PRESS
Cambridge, New York, Melbourne, Madrid, Cape Town,
Singapore, São Paulo, Delhi, Tokyo, Mexico City

Cambridge University Press
The Edinburgh Building, Cambridge CB2 8RU, UK

Published in the United States of America by
Cambridge University Press, New York

www.cambridge.org
Information on this title: www.cambridge.org/9780521514156

First published 2011
4th printing 2012

Printed in the United Kingdom at the University Press, Cambridge

A catalogue record for this publication is available from the British Library

Library of Congress Cataloging-in-Publication Data

Deep brain stimulation management / edited by William J. Marks Jr.
    p. ; cm.
    Includes bibliographical references and index.
    ISBN 978-0-521-51415-6 (Hardback)
    1. Brain stimulation–Therapeutic use.   2. Movement disorders–
Treatment.   I. Marks, William J.
    [DNLM: 1. Deep Brain Stimulation–methods.   2. Movement Disorders–
therapy. WL 390 D3114 2010]
    RC350.B72.D445 2010
    616.8′3–dc22

                                                    2010018050

ISBN 978-0-521-51415-6 Hardback

For my parents, Marlene and Bill

Contents

Contributors

Helen Bronte-Stewart, MD, MSE
Associate Professor,
Department of Neurology and
Neurological Sciences, and Director,
Stanford Movement Disorders Center,
Stanford, CA, USA

Kelly D. Foote, MD
Associate Professor,
Department of Neurosurgery, and Director,
University of Florida Movement Disorders Center,
McKnight Brain Institute, Gainesville, FL, USA

Stephen Grill, MD, PhD
Parkinson's and Movement Disorders Center of
Maryland, Elkridge, MD, USA

Ioannis U. Isaias, MD
Department of Neurology,
Mount Sinai School of Medicine,
New York, NY, USA

Lindsey Johnson, BSc
Movement Disorders Center,
Colorado Neurological Institute,
Englewood, CO, USA

Rajeev Kumar, MD, FRCPC
Medical Director,
Movement Disorders Center,
Colorado Neurological Institute,
Englewood, CO, USA

Kelly E. Lyons, PhD
Research Associate Professor of Neurology, and
Director of Research and Education,
Parkinson's Disease and Movement Disorder Center,
University of Kansas Medical Center,
Kansas City, KS, USA

William J. Marks, Jr., MD
Professor of Neurology,
University of California, San Francisco, and Director,

Parkinson's Disease Research, Education, and Clinical
Center, San Francisco Veterans Affairs Medical
Center, San Francisco, CA, USA

Erwin B. Montgomery, Jr., MD
Professor, Department of Neurology,
Division of Movement Disorders, and
Dr. Sigmund Rosen Scholar in Neurology,
University of Alabama at Birmingham, AL, USA

Michael S. Okun, MD
Associate Professor of Neurology, and Director,
University of Florida Movement Disorders Center,
McKnight Brain Institute, Gainesville, FL, USA

Jill L. Ostrem, MD
Associate Professor,
Department of Neurology, University of California,
San Francisco, and Parkinson' Disease Research,
Education, and Clinical Center,
San Francisco Veterans Affairs Medical Center,
San Francisco, CA, USA

Rajesh Pahwa, MD
Laverne and Joyce Rider
Professor of Neurology, and Director,
Parkinson's Disease and Movement Disorder Center,
University of Kansas Medical Center,
Kansas City, KS, USA

Peggie A. Smith, PA-C
Physician Assistant,
Department of Neurological Sciences,
Rush University Medical Center,
Chicago, IL, USA

Frandy Susatia, MD
Department of Neurology,
University of Florida Movement Disorders Center,
McKnight Brain Institute,
Gainesville, FL, USA

Michele Tagliati, MD
Associate Professor, and Director,
Movement Disorders,
Department of Neurology,
Cedars Sinai Medical Center,
Los Angeles, CA, USA

Leo Verhagen Metman, MD, PhD
Associate Professor of Neurological Sciences,
Rush University Medical Center,
Chicago, IL, USA

Herbert Ward, MD
Associate Professor,
Department of Psychiatry, University of Florida
Movement Disorders Center,
McKnight Brain Institute,
Gainesville, FL, USA

S. Elizabeth Zauber, MD
Assistant Professor of Clinical Neurology,
Department of Neurology,
Indiana University, Indianapolis, IN, USA

Preface

Deep brain stimulation (DBS) has evolved as an important and established treatment for movement disorders, and new indications for DBS in the treatment of neurological and psychiatric disorders are emerging. Using a fully implantable neurostimulation system, chronic DBS provides a non-destructive and reversible means of disrupting the abnormal function of brain circuits that occurs in a variety of disorders. Stimulation parameters can be programmed non-invasively to deliver the appropriate level of stimulation to the optimal anatomical region to maximize symptomatic benefits and minimize adverse effects.

Deep Brain Stimulation Management provides a concise but comprehensive and practical guide for clinicians interested in becoming involved with, or who are already involved in, using DBS for their patients.

This book was created to serve as a practical reference – a "go to" guide to be kept in the clinic and consulted in the course of managing patients being considered for or treated with DBS. *Deep Brain Stimulation Management* was designed to address in a clear manner all of the key topics pertaining to use of DBS for clinicians. Chapter 2 deals with assessing the candidacy of movement disorder patients for possible treatment with DBS. Chapter 3 focuses on the intraoperative aspects of DBS implantation surgery that are pertinent especially to the neurologist or other non-neurosurgeon clinician (though we suspect that neurosurgeons will also find this to be useful). Next,

Chapter 4 covers the neurophysiological principles underlying DBS, with the hope of demystifying the therapy and providing a foundation for the approach that clinicians undertake in programming DBS devices. Chapter 5 then covers the basic approaches to DBS programming that apply to all patients and all brain targets. Chapters 6, 7, and 8 go on to explore the specific approach to programming DBS devices and managing patients who have essential tremor, Parkinson's disease, or dystonia, respectively, with an emphasis on the unique, disease-specific issues encountered by the clinician as they care for these patients. Chapter 9 then focuses on determining whether patients have received the expected outcomes from DBS and, if not, the approach to troubleshooting suboptimal outcomes and other complications seen in the DBS patient. Finally, Chapter 10 discusses the very practical issue of how to incorporate a DBS program into clinical practice.

We have designed this book to be a valuable resource for a wide spectrum of clinicians who encounter patients with DBS, including general neurologists, movement disorder neurologists, movement disorder fellows, neurology residents, neurosurgeons, nurses, advanced practice nurses, clinical nurse specialists, nurse practitioners, physician assistants, physical therapists, and any other healthcare providers who work with patients treated with DBS.

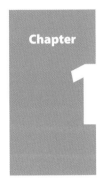

Introduction
The expanding role of deep brain stimulation

William J. Marks, Jr.

Overview

Deep brain stimulation (DBS) has evolved as an important and established treatment for movement disorders, and new indications for DBS in the treatment of neurological and psychiatric disorders are emerging. Using a fully implantable neurostimulation system, chronic DBS provides a non-destructive and reversible means of disrupting the abnormal function of thalamic and basal ganglia nuclei and their circuits that occurs in a variety of movement disorders. Stimulation parameters can be programmed non-invasively to deliver the appropriate level of stimulation to the optimal anatomical region to maximize symptomatic benefits and minimize adverse effects. The benefits of DBS compared to ablative surgery include its non-destructive nature, reversibility, and adjustability. In addition, when used bilaterally the technique does not typically produce the permanent speech, swallowing, or cognitive complications sometimes seen with ablative procedures; thus, DBS is safer for bilateral use. DBS implantation is generally safe, with serious surgical complications relatively uncommon. Adverse effects related to unintended stimulation of adjacent structures are readily reversible by altering stimulation parameters.

The DBS device and implant surgery

Deep brain stimulation uses a device with three implantable components: quadripolar brain lead(s), neurostimulator(s), and extension wire(s) (Figure 1.1).

The DBS lead, containing an array of four electrodes on its distal end, is implanted into the deep brain target using stereotactic neurosurgical techniques. Such procedures typically use image-based targeting and intraoperative physiological confirmation to accurately implant the DBS lead into the appropriate target. DBS lead implantation is often performed using local anesthesia in the awake patient to optimize the recording of physiological data during the mapping procedure, as well as to elicit the patient's report of stimulation-induced adverse effects during intraoperative test stimulation of the lead.

Following DBS lead implantation, the neurostimulator (also called an implantable pulse generator) is implanted under general anesthesia. The neurostimulator is typically placed in the subclavicular region, though it can be located elsewhere. Bilateral stimulation necessitates the implantation of two single-channel neurostimulators or one dual-channel neurostimulator. Extension wires (extensions), tunneled under the skin, connect the brain leads to the neurostimulator(s). Days to weeks after device implantation, stimulation is activated. Using the DBS programmer, the clinician can select which electrodes on the DBS lead to use to deliver stimulation, as well as the stimulation parameters themselves (including amplitude, pulse width, and rate of stimulation).

Indications for DBS

There are currently three major movement disorders for which DBS is indicated: essential tremor, Parkinson's disease, and dystonia. Deep brain stimulation at different brain targets is used to treat these disorders (Table 1.1).

Factors for success in DBS

In the opinion of many clinicians involved in the use of DBS, many patients who are good candidates for treatment with DBS fail to be referred to a DBS center

---

Table 1.1 The three major movement disorders for which deep brain stimulation is indicated

Disorder	DBS target(s)	Year of FDA approval in the USA	Comments
Essential tremor and parkinsonian tremor	Ventral intermedius nucleus of thalamus (Vim)	1997	Vim thalamic target rarely used now for parkinsonian tremor, as DBS at other targets (STN and GPi) effective for tremor suppression, as well as improvement of other cardinal PD motor features
Parkinson's disease	Subthalamic nucleus (STN) or globus pallidus internus (GPi)	2002	DBS of STN tends to be used more often for PD than DBS of GPi, though there are relative merits to both targets
Dystonia	Globus pallidus internus (GPi) or subthalamic nucleus (STN)	2003 (Humanitarian Device Exemption)	Vast majority of experience in dystonia to date is with DBS of GPi, though STN DBS is being explored

Notes: DBS, deep brain stimulation; FDA, Food and Drug Administration; PD, Parkinson's disease.

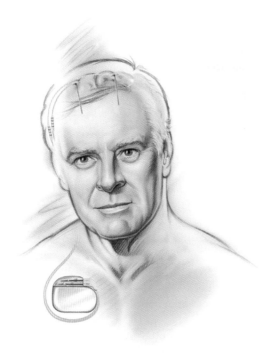

Figure 1.1 Implanted components of the deep brain stimulation (DBS) system include the DBS leads, extensions, and neurostimulator. Figure courtesy of Medtronic; used with permission.

for an evaluation to determine their suitability for this treatment option – or when they finally are referred, the patient has unnecessarily endured prolonged disability, impaired function, and compromised quality of life. Conversely, patients who are poor candidates for treatment with DBS may be referred in a "last ditch attempt to do something, when all else fails."

As experience with the clinical application of DBS has grown, several factors have emerged as vital to achieving successful outcomes for patients treated with DBS. These include:

- Appropriate patient selection, based on a multidisciplinary evaluation.
- Reasonable expectations on the part of the patient and their family regarding the outcome from DBS treatment.
- Accurate and uncomplicated implantation of the DBS leads into the appropriate anatomical target.
- Optimal programming of the DBS device, including selection and configuration of the appropriate electrode(s) on the DBS lead and choice of stimulation parameters (amplitude, pulse width, rate), in conjunction with pharmacological management.
- Adept long-term management, including management of disease progression and troubleshooting of device issues.

Note that most of these issues are non-surgical in nature. Indeed, DBS is a chronic neuromodulation therapy and not a "surgical treatment." Though it is true that expert surgical implantation of the DBS device components (especially the DBS brain leads) is necessary to achieve a successful outcome and that the surgical team is commonly involved over the long-term in the care of the patient, most of the issues to be dealt with are non-surgical in nature. Typically these issues fall under the purview of neurologists, nurses, and other non-surgeon clinicians.

DBS: a different way to think about neurological treatment

Neurologists and other clinicians who treat neurological disorders are quite familiar with pharmacological approaches to treating these conditions. The concept of using a device-based therapy to modulate brain function using electrical current may seem very foreign, however. New knowledge and skills are required to become proficient in the use of DBS. These include:

- Understanding when in the course of each patient's disease process it is appropriate to consider the use of DBS.
- Developing the processes for conducting and coordinating a multidisciplinary evaluation for DBS or aligning with an expert center to assist in this process.
- Understanding the basic neurophysiological principles underlying the use of DBS.
- Becoming familiar with the DBS device and how to optimally program it.
- Becoming comfortable with assessment of patient outcomes and determining whether patients have derived expected benefit from DBS, and how to approach troubleshooting in those who fail to achieve expected outcomes or lose benefit later.

How this book can help

In teaching clinicians around the world about the various facets of DBS for more than a decade, I have found there to be a need for a concise but comprehensive *practical* guide for clinicians interested in becoming involved with, or who are already involved in, using DBS for their patients.

Thus, this book was created to serve as a practical reference – a "go to" guide to be kept in the clinic and consulted in the course of managing patients being considered for or treated with DBS. We designed this book to address in a clear, comprehensive, and yet concise manner all of the key topics pertaining to use of DBS for clinicians. Chapter 2 deals with assessing the candidacy of movement disorder patients for possible treatment with DBS. Chapter 3 focuses on the intraoperative aspects of DBS implantation surgery that are pertinent especially to the neurologist or other non-neurosurgeon clinician (though we suspect that neurosurgeons will also find this to be useful). Next, Chapter 4 covers the neurophysiological principles underlying DBS, with the hope of demystifying the therapy and providing a foundation for the approach that clinicians undertake in programming DBS devices. Chapter 5 then covers the basic approaches to DBS programming that apply to all patients and all brain targets. Chapters 6, 7, and 8 go on to explore the specific approach to programming DBS devices and managing patients who have essential tremor, Parkinson's disease, or dystonia, respectively, with an emphasis on the unique, disease-specific issues encountered by the clinician as they care for these patients. Chapter 9 then focuses on determining whether patients have received the expected outcomes from DBS and, if not, the approach to troubleshooting suboptimal outcomes and other complications seen in the DBS patient. Finally, Chapter 10 discusses the very practical issue of how to incorporate a DBS program into clinical practice.

We hope that this book will be a valuable resource for a wide spectrum of clinicians who encounter patients with DBS, including general neurologists, movement disorder neurologists, movement disorder fellows, neurology residents, neurosurgeons, nurses, advanced practice nurses, clinical nurse specialists, nurse practitioners, physician assistants, physical therapists, and any other healthcare providers who work with patients treated with DBS.

Patient selection

When to consider deep brain stimulation for patients with Parkinson's disease, essential tremor, or dystonia

Jill L. Ostrem

Importance of patient selection

> In the use of deep brain stimulation, appropriate patient selection is a major determinant of successful postoperative outcome.

The following chapter details factors that should be considered when evaluating each patient's candidacy for deep brain stimulation (DBS). Whenever considering DBS for a patient with any type of movement disorder, the most important consideration is whether the potential risk of the DBS implant surgery is acceptable in light of the benefit that can be expected to be gained from DBS treatment. Much of the chapter will discuss this issue in detail. Having a complete understanding of what factors help predict a good outcome from DBS is essential in counseling patients, helping the clinician determine which patients are likely to realize meaningful benefit from surgery, and gauging when along the course of each patient's disease process to intervene. These factors for each individual movement disorder condition (Parkinson's disease [PD], essential tremor [ET], and dystonia) will be discussed independently. Since the potential risks associated with the surgery are similar across diagnoses (with a few exceptions), risk will be discussed for DBS in general.

Parkinson's disease

Who will benefit from surgery?

Parkinson's disease (PD) is a complex neurological disorder, with varying signs and symptoms. A patient's age of onset, specific features and distribution of motor symptomatology, rate of disease progression, and presence or absence of non-motor signs and symptoms can differ significantly and are important to take into consideration when determining if a patient is a candidate for treatment with DBS. Not all patients with PD are candidates for this therapy, but many will be.

Although surgical procedures have been employed for decades to treat PD, practices in the modern era of surgical treatment are certainly not standardized and continue to evolve as more information is obtained. Despite the absence of rigorously established guidelines for DBS candidacy, a general consensus has emerged that is useful in guiding clinical practice.

> The role of DBS is now viewed as a means of maintaining motor function before significant disability ensues – rather than being a last-resort intervention for end-stage parkinsonian patients with no other treatment options.

Indications for surgery
Certainty of diagnosis

A number of factors need to be assessed in a systematic matter to determine each patient's candidacy for treatment with DBS. This treatment is most effective and appropriate for patients with idiopathic PD, and it is generally not helpful for patients with other parkinsonian syndromes. Thus, verification of the diagnosis of idiopathic PD is the first step in assessing a patient for treatment with DBS (Table 2.1).

Not uncommonly, patients initially diagnosed with PD are later found to have another diagnosis, such as dementia with Lewy bodies (DLB), vascular parkinsonism, or a Parkinson's plus syndrome such as multiple system atrophy (MSA) or progressive supranuclear palsy (PSP). A thorough neurological history and examination focused on the patient's initial and present symptoms and signs, rate of disease progression, response to dopaminergic therapy, and presence or absence of atypical symptoms or signs can aid in confirming or refuting the diagnosis of idiopathic PD and is essential in evaluating a patient for treatment with DBS.

Identification of motor symptoms and their disability

Once the diagnosis of PD is clinically certain, clinicians should ascertain which symptoms and signs are most troublesome or disabling for the patient to determine whether those particular problems are likely to be improved by DBS.

It is now clearly recognized that DBS of the subthalamic nucleus (STN) or globus pallidus internus (GPi) improves the cardinal motor features of PD, including rigidity, tremor, bradykinesia, and in some instances disturbances of gait. In addition, a reduction in motor fluctuation is commonly seen following surgery. Patients experience quality motor function ("on" time) consistently throughout their day, with fewer episodes of troubling motor symptomatology ("off" periods) and less hyperkinetic movement (dyskinesia).[1,2]

Features of PD that appear to be less responsive to DBS include speech dysfunction, swallowing difficulty, micrographia, severe postural instability, and freezing of gait.

Postural instability and freezing of gait can be two of the most disabling symptoms, often becoming more difficult to treat pharmacologically as PD progresses. Patients with these problems are often referred for treatment with DBS when medications have failed and complicate decision making as it pertains to treatment with DBS. Severe disturbance of balance or gait unimproved by medication or that occurs when the patient is otherwise in a good state of medication-responsiveness (during the "on" period) appear to be especially resistant to improvement from

Table 2.1 Characteristic features of idiopathic Parkinson's disease[49]

- Presence of at least two of the three cardinal features of parkinsonism (rest tremor, rigidity, bradykinesia)
- Asymmetrical onset of signs/symptoms
- Substantial response to levodopa or dopamine agonist
- Absence of features suggesting alternative diagnoses:
  - Prominent postural instability in the first three years after symptom onset
  - Freezing phenomena early in the first three years
  - Hallucinations unrelated to medication in the first three years of disease
  - Dementia preceding motor symptoms or in the first year
  - Supranuclear gaze palsy
  - Upper motor neuron signs on examination
  - Severe, symptomatic dysautonomia unrelated to medications
  - Documentation of a condition known to produce parkinsonism and plausibly connected to the patient's symptoms

DBS. When these symptoms occur in the "off" period alone, some benefit may still be obtained from DBS, but in our experience the effect may not be sustained over time (Table 2.2).

Though not well studied, many non-motor manifestations of PD (e.g., cognitive dysfunction, dysautonomia) do not appear to benefit from DBS. Recognizing the non-motor factors that contribute to each patient's disability and the extent to which the patient's most troubling symptoms respond to DBS will help identify those patients who will experience the greatest benefit from treatment with DBS. Table 2.3 lists questions that can be helpful in assessing the presence and extent of various motor symptoms preoperatively.

From a careful patient history one can develop an appreciation for the level of disability experienced by each patient. In order to justify the potential risk of surgical implantation of DBS leads, patients should be at a stage in their PD in which they are experiencing significant disability. Determining what constitutes significant disability is subjective and should be individualized for each patient.

> The goal is to intervene, if possible, when the patient reaches a stage where the daily burden of parkinsonian motor symptomatology just begins to cause significant interference with daily function, occupational activities, important leisure time pursuits, and/or basic activities of daily living.

Table 2.2 Symptom response to deep brain stimulation for Parkinson's disease

Symptom	Improves	Generally does not improve
Tremor	X	
Bradykinesia	X	
Rigidity	X	
Dyskinesia	X	
Motor fluctuations	X	
Hypophonic speech		X
Dysphagia		X
Micrographia		X
Freezing of gait, especially if occurring in the "on" state		X
Balance abnormalities of significant extent		X
Cognitive dysfunction		X
Dysautonomia		X

A useful tool in gauging daily function is the motor fluctuation diary, a chart in which the patient records their level of motor function periodically throughout their day (Appendix A). Typically patients are asked to rate their motor function every 30–60 minutes during wakefulness as to whether they are "off" (slow and/or experiencing other troublesome symptoms), "on" (functioning reasonably well), or "on with troublesome dyskinesia" (experiencing excessive, involuntary movement that impedes function). Patients are also asked to indicate when medications were taken, allowing the clinician interpretation of relationships between motor function and medication timing. Such "real time" ratings by patients and their family members provide extremely helpful information in understanding the cumulative quantity and patterns of motor disability throughout each patient's day.

Table 2.3 Questions to help understand Parkinson's disease motor symptomatology and disability

1. What are the symptoms from your Parkinson's disease that bother you the most, beginning with the most troublesome problem, in order of severity?
2. Do you have tremor or shaking, and how much of a problem is it for you?
3. Do you have rigidity or muscle stiffness, and how much of a problem is it for you?
4. Do you have slowness of movement or difficulty initiating movement, and how much of a problem is it for you?
5. Do you have trouble with walking, and how much of a problem is it for you?
6. Do you have problems with balance, and how much of a problem is it for you?
7. Do you experience freezing of gait? Do you feel like your feet get glued to the ground? If so, when does this occur?
8. Do you fall? If so, why and how often?
9. During what percent of your waking day are you "off," that is, experiencing significant symptoms from your Parkinson's disease, despite taking your medication?
10. How would you describe the most severe "off" state on a typical day?
11. During what percent of your waking day do you experience troublesome dyskinesia, that is, excessive and uncontrollable movement that bothers you?
12. What activities were you previously able to perform that are now difficult or impossible due to your Parkinson's disease?

Some surgical research protocols require that patients experience a minimum amount (e.g., three or more hours) of cumulative "off" and/or dyskinetic time each day to justify DBS implant surgery.

Tools useful to document the extent of dyskinesia include the Unified Parkinson's Disease Rating Scale (UPDRS) Part IVa (dyskinesia) score (Appendix B), the Abnormal Involuntary Movement Scale (AIMS) (Appendix C), or the Rush Dyskinesia Scale.[3] To assess health-related quality of life, the Parkinson's Disease Questionnaire (PDQ-39) can also be used (Appendix D).[4]

Table 2.4 Strategies for optimizing pharmacological treatment of motor symptoms in Parkinson's disease before proceeding with deep brain stimulation

1. Administer immediate release levodopa at the appropriate dose and frequency tailored to the patient's wake/sleep, meal, and activity schedule (note that in advanced patients, controlled-release preparations of levodopa are often less consistent in their effect). This is typically five or more times a day

2. Use a dopamine agonist at appropriate doses in conjunction with levodopa as tolerated; if one agonist is ineffective or poorly tolerated, consider a trial of another agonist

3. Use a catechol-O-methyltransferase (COMT) inhibitor to maximize the duration of effect from levodopa

4. Use a monoamine oxidase B (MAO-B) inhibitor to increase "on-time"

5. Use an anti-cholinergic medication if the patient has severe tremor or dystonic dyskinesia

6. Use amantadine up to three times a day to treat troublesome dyskinesia

7. Consider the use of injectable apomorphine to rescue patients from severe "off" periods

Status of pharmacological treatment

Since DBS suppresses symptoms but is not thought to alter disease progression, DBS is generally used to control symptoms only when pharmacotherapy fails to provide adequate, consistent relief of symptoms. To deem medication treatment sufficiently ineffective before proceeding to DBS surgery, one needs to ensure the patient's medication regimen has been optimized for their particular symptoms. The patient's current and past PD medications and dosing schedule should be carefully reviewed. Ensuring that reasonable pharmacological treatment options have been undertaken to improve control of symptoms, motor fluctuations, and dyskinesia is critical. If not already undertaken, the strategies listed in Table 2.4 can be considered in an attempt to optimize pharmacological treatment before considering DBS. Most of these strategies can be employed relatively quickly to determine whether symptoms can be brought under adequate control and DBS surgery can be deferred or not. In some patients, medications are poorly tolerated. Proceeding to surgery earlier, without exhausting all medication options, may be appropriate in this situation.

Extent of dopaminergic responsiveness

The degree to which a patient is responsive to dopaminergic medication, particularly levodopa, generally predicts how responsive motor symptoms will be to DBS.[5] Levodopa responsiveness can sometimes be inferred from a careful history, but having objective confirmation of levodopa responsiveness and its extent can be helpful when evaluating a patient for treatment with DBS. The most widely used scale to assess motor signs in patients with PD is the motor subscale (Part III) of the UPDRS (Table 2.5 and Appendix B).[6] Many clinicians assess the UPDRS III score with the patient in their most symptomatic ("off") state and then again once the patient has responded to their anti-parkinsonian medication and has achieved their best motor function ("on" state). This is practically achieved by assessing the patient in the morning, following cessation of anti-parkinsonian medication for about 12 hours overnight, and then again after the patient has ingested their usual morning dose of medication (with or without extra levodopa) and derived a good response. Evaluation of the patient in the "off" state provides an instructive glimpse into the patient's motor symptoms and associated disability at its most severe (not often appreciated in a routine office visit). It also allows for an objective comparison of the "off" and "on" UPDRS III scores, confirming the degree of responsiveness to dopaminergic medication, and can help gauge which symptoms will likely respond to DBS and to what extent. The minimal degree of improvement required after a dopaminergic challenge for a patient to be considered a candidate for DBS is not well established, although many clinicians desire at least a 30% improvement in UPDRS III score and a minimum UPDRS III score of 30/108 in the "off" state.[7] The Core Assessment Program for the Surgical Interventional Therapies in Parkinson's Disease (CAPSIT-PD) recommends a 33% improvement in the UPDRS III subscore or greater before recommending surgery.[8] Rarely is DBS surgery offered to patients who do not demonstrate at least a 30% improvement. By performing these measures, one also derives information helpful in educating the patient and family about which symptoms are most likely to respond to DBS.

> As discussed earlier, symptoms and signs resistant to levodopa will likely be resistant to DBS, with the notable exception of medication-resistant tremor.

7

Table 2.5 Unified Parkinson's Disease Rating Scale (UPDRS) Motor Subscale (Part III)

18. Speech
    - □ (0) Normal
    - □ (1) Slight loss of expression, diction, and/or volume
    - □ (2) Monotone, slurred but understandable; moderately impaired
    - □ (3) Marked impairment, difficult to understand
    - □ (4) Unintelligible

19. Facial expression
    - □ (0) Normal
    - □ (1) Minimal hypomimia, could be normal "Poker Face"
    - □ (2) Slight but definitely abnormal diminution of facial expression
    - □ (3) Moderate hypomimia; lips parted some of the time
    - □ (4) Masked or fixed facies with severe or complete loss of facial expression; lips part ¼ inch or more

20. Tremor at rest (head, upper and lower extremities)
    - (0) Absent
    - (1) Slight and infrequently present
    - (2) Mild in amplitude and persistent. Or moderate in amplitude, but only intermittently present
    - (3) Moderate in amplitude and present most of the time
    - (4) Marked in amplitude and present most of the time

    20a. Face: □ (0) □ (1) □ (2) □ (3) □ (4)

    20b. Right upper extremity:
    □ (0) □ (1) □ (2) □ (3) □ (4)

    20c. Left upper extremity:
    □ (0) □ (1) □ (2) □ (3) □ (4)

    20d. Right lower extremity:
    □ (0) □ (1) □ (2) □ (3) □ (4)

    20e. Left lower extremity:
    □ (0) □ (1) □ (2) □ (3) □ (4)

21. Action or postural tremor of hands
    - (0) Absent
    - (1) Slight; present with action
    - (2) Moderate in amplitude, present with action
    - (3) Moderate in amplitude with posture holding as well as action
    - (4) Marked in amplitude; interferes with feeding

    21a. Right: □ (0) □ (1) □ (2) □ (3) □ (4)
    21b. Left: □ (0) □ (1) □ (2) □ (3) □ (4)

22. Rigidity (Judged on passive movement of major jobs with subject relaxed in sitting position. Cogwheeling to be ignored)
    - (0) Absent
    - (1) Slight or detectable only when activated by mirror or other movements
    - (2) Mild to moderate
    - (3) Marked, but full range of motion easily achieved
    - (4) Severe, range of motion achieved with difficulty

    22a. Neck: □ (0) □ (1) □ (2) □ (3) □ (4)

    22b. Right upper extremity:
    □ (0) □ (1) □ (2) □ (3) □ (4)

    22c. Left upper extremity:
    □ (0) □ (1) □ (2) □ (3) □ (4)

    22d. Right lower extremity:
    □ (0) □ (1) □ (2) □ (3) □ (4)

    22e. Left lower extremity:
    □ (0) □ (1) □ (2) □ (3) □ (4)

23. Finger taps (Subject taps thumb with index finder in rapid succession)
    - (0) Normal
    - (1) Mild slowing and/or reduction in amplitude
    - (2) Moderately impaired. Definite and early fatiguing. May have occasional arrests in movement
    - (3) Severely impaired. Frequent hesitation in initiating movements or arrests in ongoing movement
    - (4) Can barely perform the task

    23a. Right: □ (0) □ (1) □ (2) □ (3) □ (4)
    23b. Left: □ (0) □ (1) □ (2) □ (3) □ (4)

24. Hand movements (Subject opens and closes hands in rapid succession)
    - (0) Normal
    - (1) Mild slowing and/or reduction in amplitude
    - (2) Moderately impaired. Definite and early fatiguing. May have occasional arrests in movement

Table 2.5 (*cont.*)

(3) Severely impaired. Frequent hesitation in initiating movements or arrests in ongoing movement

(4) Can barely perform task

24a. Right: ☐ (0) ☐ (1) ☐ (2) ☐ (3) ☐ (4)

24b. Left: ☐ (0) ☐ (1) ☐ (2) ☐ (3) ☐ (4)

25. Rapid alternating movements of hands (Pronation–supination movements of hands, vertically and horizontally, with as large an amplitude as possible, both hands simultaneously)

(0) Normal

(1) Mild slowing and/or reduction in amplitude

(2) Moderately impaired. Definite and early fatiguing. May have occasional arrests in movement

(3) Severely impaired. Frequent hesitation in initiating movements or arrests in ongoing movement

(4) Can barely perform task

25a. Right: ☐ (0) ☐ (1) ☐ (2) ☐ (3) ☐ (4)

25b. Left: ☐ (0) ☐ (1) ☐ (2) ☐ (3) ☐ (4)

26. Leg agility (Subject taps heel on the ground in rapid succession picking up entire leg. Amplitude should be at least 3 inches)

(0) Normal

(1) Mild slowing and/or reduction in amplitude

(2) Moderately impaired. Definite and early fatiguing. May have occasional arrests in movement

(3) Severely impaired. Frequent hesitation in initiating movements or arrests in ongoing movement

(4) Can barely perform the task

26a. Right: ☐ (0) ☐ (1) ☐ (2) ☐ (3) ☐ (4)

26b. Left: ☐ (0) ☐ (1) ☐ (2) ☐ (3) ☐ (4)

27. Arising from chair (Subject attempts to rise from a straight-backed chair, with arms folded across chest)

☐ (0) Normal

☐ (1) Slow; or may need more than one attempt

☐ (2) Pushes self up from arms of seat

☐ (3) Tends to fall back and may need to try more than one time, but can get up without help

☐ (4) Unable to arise without help

28. Posture

☐ (0) Normal

☐ (1) Not quite erect, slightly stooped

☐ (2) Moderately stooped posture, definitely abnormal; can be slightly leaning to one side

☐ (3) Severely stooped posture with kyphosis; can be moderately leaning to one side

☐ (4) Marked flexion with extreme abnormality of posture

29. Gait

☐ (0) Normal

☐ (1) Walks slowly, may shuffle with short steps, but no festination (hastening steps) or propulsion

☐ (2) Walks with difficulty, but requires little or no assistance; may have festination, short steps, or propulsion

☐ (3) Severe disturbance of gait, requiring assistance

☐ (4) Cannot walk at all, even with assistance

30. Postural stability (Response to sudden, strong posterior displacement produced by pull on shoulders while subject erect with eyes open and feet slightly apart. Subject is prepared)

☐ (0) Normal

☐ (1) Retropulsion, but recovers unaided

☐ (2) Absence of postural response; would fall if not caught by examiner

☐ (3) Very unstable, tends to lose balance spontaneously

☐ (4) Unable to stand without assistance

31. Body bradykinesia and hypokinesia (Combining slowness, hesitancy, decreased arm swing, small amplitude, and poverty of motion in general)

☐ (0) None

☐ (1) Minimal slowness, giving movement a deliberate character; could be normal for some persons. Possibly reduced amplitude

☐ (2) Mild degree of slowness and poverty of movement, which is definitely abnormal. Alternatively, some reduced amplitude

☐ (3) Moderate slowness, poverty or small amplitude of movement

☐ (4) Marked slowness, poverty or small amplitude of movement

Source: The Movement Disorder Society (see: http://www.movementdisorders.org/publications/rating_scales/)

We also find that videotaping the patient's preoperative examination during the "off" and "on" UPDRS III assessments provides a useful visual record of baseline motor dysfunction, which can later be reviewed postoperatively to appreciate treatment response.

Cognitive status

> A clear understanding of the patient's cognitive function is important when considering candidacy for DBS.

Dementia is common in patients with PD, with the prevalence increasing with advanced age and disease progression.[9] Most clinicians do not offer DBS to patients with bona fide dementia. The presence of dementia in a patient suggests that they have more widespread disease, which may be a marker for less robust motor response to DBS. Additionally, the presence of dementia produces practical obstacles to achieving optimal outcomes. Patients with dementia have difficulty tolerating and cooperating with the awake surgical procedures typically employed. Patients with dementia also have difficulty accurately observing and articulating their symptoms, making adjustment of DBS parameters and medications more difficult. Finally, patients with pre-existing dementia may experience a worsening of their cognitive status following DBS surgery, leading to more disability.[10–12]

To screen for dementia, a Mini Mental Status Exam (MMSE) can be performed. It is generally accepted that a MMSE score of ≤ 24 is an indicator of poor candidacy for DBS surgery.[7] More recently, the Montreal Cognitive Assessment (MoCA) has been suggested as a more appropriate cognitive screening test, as it tests a wider range of cognitive domains than the MMSE and can detect deficiencies earlier in the course of PD (Appendix E).[13,14] Many clinicians at experienced DBS centers evaluate all patients being considered for DBS with a battery of neurocognitive tests preoperatively. Certainly, if the history or screening examination raises concerns about a patient's cognitive status, formal neuropsychological testing should be performed. Patients with PD can develop cognitive deficits in areas of executive functioning, visuospatial processing, attention and set shifting, and memory function. In the neurocognitive testing battery, it is important to include measures of general cognitive functioning, such as the Mattis Dementia Rating Scale (MDRS); measures of

executive functioning and attention, such as verbal fluency tests, paced auditory serial addition tests, or the Wisconsin Card Sorting Test; measures of short- and long-term memory function; measures of visuospatial function; and measures of language function. In some instances, results from neuropsychological testing may reveal a pattern of dementia that is more compatible with Alzheimer's disease, diffuse Lewy body disease, or PSP, offering evidence against the pursuit of DBS for that patient. Some clinicians exclude patients based on an MDRS total score of ≤ 120–$130/144$[7,8] or use a rejection criterion of an MDRS total score two or more standard deviations below the age-adjusted mean normal score, or the criterion of two or more (out of five) subtest scores that lie beyond two standard deviations.

Mood and psychotic symptoms

Patients with PD are prone to depression, anxiety, and psychotic symptoms, including hallucinations and delusions. These symptoms can be a direct result of the disease process or exacerbated by medications used to control the symptoms of PD. The prevalence of depression in PD patients ranges from 20 to 50%,[15] with the majority of these patients meeting criteria for anxiety as well.

The literature is conflicted on the effect of DBS on mood. Some studies suggest improvement in mood after surgery[16,17]; however, a growing body of literature suggests that, in some individuals, depression and anxiety can worsen after DBS surgery.[18,19] Although there is no clear evidence that the presence of pre-existing mood disorder increases the risk of postoperative disturbance in mood, it seems reasonable to assume that before proceeding with surgery, mood disorders should be identified and effectively treated.

> Furthermore, offering DBS surgery to patients with severe pre-existing depression or anxiety that does not adequately respond to pharmacological treatment may not be advisable.

The Geriatric Depression Scale – Short Form has been suggested by specialists as a useful tool for screening for depression in PD (Appendix F).[20] Also the Beck Depression Inventory (BDI), the Hamilton Depression Rating Scale, and the

Montgomery and Asberg Depression Rating Scale (MADRS) have been recommended to assess depression by the American Academy of Neurology.[21] In our center, if a patient has a score of >15 on the BDI, then surgery is generally not recommended. The CAPSIT-PD recommends a score ranging from 7–19 on the MADRS as an exclusion criterion.[8]

Parkinson's disease patients referred for surgery are also at greater risk for psychotic symptoms, as they usually have relatively advanced disease and are being treated with moderate to high doses of medications that have the potential to cause adverse psychiatric effects. Patients with active hallucinations or delusions may be at increased risk for psychiatric complications after DBS surgery. A wide range of psychiatric symptoms has been described following STN DBS surgery, including hallucinations, severe psychosis, mania, and impulsivity.[17] Many times these symptoms occur in the immediate postoperative period, when patients are hospitalized, and are transient. Cases of persistent postoperative behavioral disturbance have been reported, though, and these may be more likely to occur in patients who are prone to these problems preoperatively.[10]

> Thus, patients with significant, unresolved psychotic symptoms should not undergo DBS surgery.[10,22]

In many instances, reduction of anti-parkinsonian medication or addition of an atypical antipsychotic agent can improve these symptoms, with the patient then able to proceed with DBS surgery.

> Certainly, if a patient's psychotic symptoms are mild and clearly medication-induced, then treatment with DBS may be beneficial, since postoperative reduction in medication, and its associated adverse effects, is often possible.

Upper age limit

Whether there is an upper age limit above which DBS surgery should no longer be offered is a topic of debate. Findings of only modest motor improvement in older patients after STN DBS surgery have been reported.[5,23] Others have found an increased

incidence of cognitive dysfunction in older patients after DBS surgery.[10] Older patients may tolerate surgery less well and may be more susceptible to transient postoperative confusion, especially after bilateral STN DBS surgery. Several experienced DBS centers prefer to stage DBS brain lead implantation surgeries by several weeks to months in older patients, performing only one DBS lead implant into one hemisphere at a time to minimize postoperative confusion and aid in recovery time. We and others, however, have found no difference in postoperative outcomes in patients with advanced age, providing these patients are carefully selected and exhibit a robust response to a dopaminergic challenge.[24–26]

> We typically do not exclude patients from surgery based on age alone. If older patients experience severe motor fluctuations, dyskinesia, a good response to levodopa, no signs of dementia or major psychiatric disturbance, and are in good general health, we will offer treatment with DBS.

Unilateral versus bilateral treatment

The ability to safely provide bilateral treatment with DBS has led to this treatment being used bilaterally in the majority of PD patients who experience bilateral appendicular and/or axial motor symptoms. In moderately advanced patients with PD, bilateral treatment with subthalamic or pallidal DBS provides incremental benefit over unilateral treatment and allows for a greater reduction in postoperative medication requirements. Unilateral DBS used in patients with bilateral symptoms generally provides incomplete benefit and can result in more challenging postoperative management. Certainly, in patients with unilateral or strongly asymmetric motor symptoms, contralateral unilateral surgical intervention with DBS is appropriate.

Previous surgery for PD

In general, previous ablative surgery does not exclude the possibility of additional surgical intervention. In a patient with a previous unilateral pallidotomy who continues to experience contralateral benefit but now requires treatment on the opposite side, pallidal DBS on the opposite side of the brain can be used. Alternatively, if the benefits from the previous pallidotomy have waned, bilateral STN DBS can be employed with excellent benefit.[27] Patients with a previous thalamotomy can also be successfully treated with bilateral STN or GPi DBS.

Surgical brain target selection

The surgical treatment of choice today for most patients with PD is DBS. The best location for stimulation, however, remains controversial. Both the STN and GPi have been studied extensively as target locations for DBS, and both have been shown to treat the cardinal motor features of PD. Comparative studies to date and a meta-analysis of reports concerning DBS of the STN or of the GPi have shown no statistically significant difference in the motor improvement provided by these treatments.[28] A large-scale, multicenter, prospective randomized study sponsored by the Department of Veterans Affairs Cooperative Studies Program and the National Institute of Neurological Diseases and Stroke comparing bilateral STN and GPi DBS has recently been completed. The findings from this landmark study are helping to clarify numerous issues concerning the use of DBS at the two targets.[29]

In many centers DBS of the STN is the default surgical target. Subthalamic nucleus stimulation may currently offer several advantages over pallidal stimulation. These include the larger scope of published experience with DBS of the STN, the greater familiarity that many neurosurgeons have in mapping and operating upon this target, and the suggestion from clinical practice that postoperative medication reduction is greater in patients treated at this target.[30] Conversely, pallidal stimulation may offer some advantages over subthalamic stimulation. Some have suggested that GPi DBS provides a direct anti-dyskinetic effect on levodopa-induced dyskinesia, allowing medication levels to be maintained to help treat symptoms in a synergistic manner.[31] Additionally, cognitive, mood, and behavior abnormalities may be less prevalent in patients treated with GPi DBS compared with those receiving STN stimulation, though this remains to be proven.[32]

Deep brain stimulation at the thalamic target (specifically, the ventral intermediate nucleus of the thalamus) is effective in suppressing contralateral parkinsonian tremor but does not address other motor symptoms.[33,34] In contrast, DBS of either the STN or of the GPi can provide effective tremor

Table 2.6 Summary of generally accepted criteria of deep brain stimulation candidacy for treatment of Parkinson's disease

Inclusion criteria	Exclusion criteria
Diagnosis of idiopathic PD	Serious surgical co-morbidities
Disabling or troubling motor symptoms, including motor fluctuations or dyskinesia, despite optimized pharmacological treatment	Uncontrolled psychiatric illness, including anxiety and mood disorder (BDI > 15)
Robust motor response (other than tremor) to levodopa (>30% improvement of UPDRS III score)	Dementia (MMSE $\leq$ 24, MDRS $\leq$ 130)
Clear understanding of risks and realistic expectations from surgery	Preoperative MRI with extensive white matter changes or severe cerebral atrophy

Notes: BDI, Beck Depression Inventory; MDRS, Mattis Dementia Rating Scale; MMSE, Mini Mental Status Examination; PD, Parkinson's disease; UPDRS III, Unified Parkinson's Disease Rating Scale, Part III (Motor Subscale).

control while simultaneously improving other parkinsonian motor symptoms, diminishing motor fluctuation, and suppressing dyskinesia. Thus, even in those patients with PD who predominantly manifest tremor as their main source of disability, basal ganglia targets seem to be preferable to the thalamic target in many of these instances (Table 2.6).

Essential tremor
Certainty of diagnosis of ET

When considering a patient with ET for DBS, it is once again important to make sure the patient meets clinical criteria for the diagnosis of ET as a first step. It is estimated that 30–50% of patients with ET are commonly misdiagnosed with PD or other tremor disorders.[35] Essential tremor may be a heterogeneous group of disorders caused by different pathogenic mechanisms.[36] The core and secondary criteria developed to help facilitate a practical approach to the diagnosis of ET are helpful to review (Table 2.7).

It is important to make an accurate diagnosis, as other causes of tremor may not respond to DBS

Table 2.7 Features characteristic of idiopathic essential tremor[50]

Core criteria

- Bilateral action tremor of the hands and forearms (but not rest tremor)
- Absence of other neurological signs with the exception of the cogwheel phenomenon
- May have isolated head tremor with no signs of dystonia

Secondary criteria

- Long duration (>3 years)
- Positive family history
- Beneficial response to alcohol

Table 2.8 Diagnostic "red flags" indicating tremor disorder other than essential tremor and the most likely diagnoses[50,51]

"Red flags"	Most likely differential diagnosis
Unilateral tremor, leg tremor, rigidity, bradykinesia, rest tremor	Parkinson's disease
Gait disturbance	Parkinson's disease, cerebellar tremor
Focal tremor	Dystonic tremor
Isolated head tremor with abnormal posture (head tilt or turning)	Cervical dystonia
Sudden or rapid onset	Psychogenic tremor, toxic tremor
Current drug treatment that might cause or exacerbate tremor	Drug-induced tremor or toxic tremor

and may have other treatments available to improve symptoms. Table 2.8 lists common red flags to consider when evaluating a patient with tremor.

Identification of severity of tremor and related disability

The severity of the tremor in patients with ET varies widely. Although some patients have only a fine, low amplitude postural tremor in their hands, others will have severe tremor. Most patients considering DBS will be experiencing moderate to severe disability from the tremor. In general, when the tremor impairs feeding, using a spoon, drinking from a cup, writing, typing, or hygiene; interferes with occupational motor tasks; or leads to social isolation then DBS should be considered.

Status of pharmacological treatment

Before considering DBS surgery, it is important to review medications that patients have been prescribed for their tremor. The two most effective and well-studied medications for ET, propranolol and primidone, are effective in 30–70% of patients.[37,38] The beta-blocker propranolol is usually dosed between 60 and 800 mg per day, but its use can be associated with hypotension, bradycardia, impotence, drowsiness, confusion, headache, and exercise intolerance.[37] Primidone can be dosed at 25–750 mg per day, but up to 20% of patients cannot tolerate this medication (even initiating the drug at very low doses) because of drowsiness or unsteadiness.[39] Other less well-studied oral agents that can be used to treat ET include other beta-adrenergic receptor antagonists (atenolol, nadolol, sotalol), benzodiazepines, topiramate, and gabapentin.[38] These medications have varying effectiveness and may be worth exploring, but delay in referring for ventral intermedius (Vim) DBS should be minimized, given the robust effectiveness of this intervention.

Unilateral versus bilateral treatment

It is also important to determine if the patient will sufficiently benefit from a single unilateral Vim DBS implant, or if bilateral DBS will be necessary to achieve adequate tremor control. In some patients, achieving tremor control in the dominant hand alone will improve functioning enough and can avoid the additional surgical risk of placing the contralateral brain lead. In patients who require both hands to be free of tremor for effective functioning, bilateral DBS will be needed. In this case patients should be counseled that the likelihood of developing mild speech difficulties or balance abnormalities after bilateral Vim thalamic DBS lead placement is increased compared to unilateral treatment.

Dystonia
Indications and patient evaluation

Determining which dystonia patients are candidates for DBS can be more challenging than making this determination for patients with PD or ET. Dystonia is a heterogeneous group of disorders with multiple etiologies and varying clinical presentations. Currently, there are few controlled studies looking at predictors of outcome following DBS in these patients. What is known is that some forms of dystonia will respond more favorably than others. Characterizing and classifying the type of dystonia as much as possible is useful in determining who should be considered for DBS surgery.

Clarification of diagnosis

Patients referred for DBS surgery for treatment of dystonia should undergo a detailed history of illness and physical examination to determine the dystonia type and possible etiology. Dystonia is classified as generalized when it affects the trunk and at least one leg, segmental when it affects two adjoining body regions, focal when it affects one body region, or hemidystonia when it affects one side of the body. The body distribution affected by the dystonia helps to shed light on the possible underlying etiology. Understanding the cause (if one can be identified) of the dystonia symptoms is very important. When no underlying cause of the patient's dystonia can be determined or if the dystonia is from a known *DYT1* mutation, then dystonia is considered primary. When the dystonia is a result of a known cause or the result of an underlying brain injury, it is considered secondary. Examples of secondary dystonia are presented in Table 2.9.

> In general, patients with primary dystonia tend to respond much better to DBS than patients with secondary forms of dystonia.[40]

Most clinical trials have studied patients with primary generalized dystonia, but there is also a growing literature for the use of DBS in refractory primary focal and primary segmental dystonia.

> An exception is tardive dystonia; though considered a secondary dystonia, patients with this type of dystonia tend to respond very well to DBS.[41]

To help confirm whether a patient has primary or secondary dystonia, brain imaging (MRI if possible)

Table 2.9 Secondary dystonias: a large and diverse group of disorders

Acquired structural lesions

- Perinatal injury, kernicterus, infarcts, hemorrhage, brain infection, trauma, anoxia, toxin exposure, multiple sclerosis, and brain tumors

Metabolic or heredodegenerative disorders

- Wilson's disease
- Parkinsonian syndromes
  - Parkinson's disease, juvenile parkinsonism, multisystem atrophy, corticobasal degeneration, progressive supranuclear palsy
- Globus pallidus degenerations
- Pantothenate kinase deficiency due to *PANK2* mutations
- Familial basal ganglia calcifications
- Huntington's disease
- Spinocerebellar degeneration
- Lysosomal storage disorders
- Organic aminoacidurias (gluteric aciduria, propionic academia, and methylmalonic acidura)
- Mitochondrial disorders
- Neuroacanthocytosis
- Lesch–Nyhan syndrome
- Ataxia-telangiectasia

Tardive dystonia

should be performed to determine structural abnormalities underlying secondary causes of dystonia. In cases of childhood-onset generalized dystonia, the diagnosis of dopa-responsive dystonia (*DYT5* dystonia, also called Segawa's disease) should be excluded with a trial of levodopa, as this disorder can mimic idiopathic generalized dystonia, is treatable, and is exquisitely responsive to treatment with levodopa, obviating the need for DBS.

Documentation of dystonia

Before undergoing DBS surgery, a detailed videotaped clinical evaluation should be performed that includes standardized dystonia rating scales, if possible. Establishing a clear baseline of symptom distribution and severity is important. The most commonly used rating scale to measure the severity and disability from generalized dystonia is the Burke–Fahn–Marsden Dystonia Rating Scale (BFMDRS) (Appendix G).[42,43] This scale is composed of a movement scale (based on an objective motor exam) and a disability scale (based on a patient interview). The 120-point movement scale rates the severity of dystonia in 9 body regions, taking into account both the severity and frequency of the dystonic movements. This scale has shown excellent inter-rater reliability and has emerged as a preferred rating scale for generalized dystonia.[42,43] The most commonly used rating scale for cervical dystonia is the Toronto Western Spasmodic Torticollis Rating Scale (TWSTRS),[44] an 85-point scale with subscores for dystonia severity, functional disability, and pain (Appendix H). For both scales, a higher score indicates more severe dystonia. Although these rating scales result in objective outcome measures, they are limited in measuring fixed versus mobile dystonia and complex movements. Performing videotaped exams is also helpful to provide clear documentation of the dystonia.

Status of pharmacological treatment

As with patients with PD or ET, it is important that patients are offered DBS only after they have failed to adequately respond to reasonable attempts to control the dystonia with medical management. Patients with primary generalized dystonia should have tried treatment with anticholinergic, antiepileptic, and benzodiazepine medications, as well as baclofen. Dystonia of this type, however, is typically not very responsive to oral medications, and the medications often produce intolerable adverse effects. Juvenile-onset dystonia is an exception, though, since patients with this disorder can respond favorably to anticholinergic medications and tend to tolerate such treatment. In patients with focal or segmental dystonia, treatment failure with similar medications should be reviewed. Additionally, if patients fail to achieve adequate symptom relief after botulinum toxin injections with appropriate muscle selection and dosing, DBS should be considered.

Predictive factors

Few studies have assessed predictors of outcome in dystonia patients undergoing DBS. One recent study found that primary generalized dystonia patients with shorter duration of disease had better outcomes but noted no predictive value of age of dystonia onset, age at time of DBS surgery, severity of disease, *DYT1* status, or the presence of phasic or tonic dystonic movements.[45] The influence of these factors on adult-onset focal/segmental dystonia remains unknown. It does appear that patients who are DBS candidates should undergo surgery prior to the onset of fixed skeletal deformities, which if present may limit functional improvement even when dystonia symptoms are ameliorated.[45,46]

Assessment of disability from dystonia

It is generally agreed that patients undergoing DBS for dystonia should be experiencing some level of disability from their dystonia. The degree of disability may vary across patients and may be related to impaired movements, pain, social isolation, or often a combination of all of these factors. Both the BFMDRS and the TWSTRS have disability subscales that are helpful in documenting the level of disability, which may help to support moving forward with DBS surgery.

Neuropsychological and psychiatric assessments

Little is known about the impact of cognitive status, mood, and psychotic symptoms in dystonia patients and how much these factors should weigh in determining candidacy for DBS. Most patients with primary dystonia will not have significant cognitive dysfunction or psychotic symptoms; however, it is not uncommon to see significant depression or anxiety in this patient population. Having a neuropsychologist or psychiatrist evaluate the patient and identify significant mood symptoms to treat before surgery is generally recommended.

Target choice

Traditionally, patients with dystonia have been treated with DBS of the GPi. Almost all dystonia DBS outcome studies reflect patients treated with DBS at the GPi target. Patients who are appropriate candidates for treatment with DBS who have primary generalized dystonia realize excellent outcomes with GPi DBS. Limited reports of thalamic DBS in dystonia have reported disappointing results. It is unclear at this time if other brain targets, such as the STN, might also be helpful in treating dystonia, and STN DBS is currently being explored for treating some dystonia subtypes.

Table 2.10 Expected outcome after globus pallidus internus (GPi) deep brain stimulation (DBS) based on dystonia subtype[40]

Dystonia classification	Typical expected outcome
Juvenile onset primary generalized (with or without *DYT1* mutation)	50–70% improvement in BFMDRS movement score
Adult onset cervical	45–70% improvement in TWSTRS severity subscore
Adult onset cranial/cervical dystonia	45–80% improvement in BFMDRS movement score
Tardive dystonia	35–75% improvement in BFMDRS movement score
Secondary dystonia	10–20% improvement in BFMDRS movement score

Notes: BFMDRS, Burke–Fahn–Marsden Dystonia Rating Scale; TWSTRS, Toronto Western Spasmodic Torticollis Rating Scale.

Table 2.11 Key factors in determining patient candidacy for a rechargeable neurostimulator

1. Does the patient have the cognitive function required to ensure the battery is properly recharged? Will they as the disease progresses?
2. Is there patient interest?
3. Does the patient have a caregiver who could offer support if needed?
4. Does the patient have a high expected battery consumption that would justify implanting a rechargeable device?
5. Does the patient have the manual dexterity to operate the recharging system effectively?

Counseling patients on expected DBS surgical outcome

Once a dystonia patient has been properly evaluated and screened for DBS, it is important to counsel the patient on the degree of expected improvement in symptoms with DBS treatment. Patients with childhood/juvenile-onset primary generalized dystonia generally have the best outcome, with improvements of 50–70% as measured by the BFMDRS movement score commonly achieved. Adult-onset cranial/cervical and tardive dystonia patients can expect to improve 35–80% as measured by standardized dystonia scales. Secondary dystonia typically responds more modestly (10–20% reduction in dystonia scores), though this level of improvement can be clinically meaningful.[40] These estimates should only be used as a general guide, and the emphasis in counseling should be on the wide range of outcomes after DBS surgery in patients with dystonia (Table 2.10).

Factors relevant to PD, ET, and dystonia patients considering DBS surgery

Surgical risk

The two most important risks of surgery are hemorrhagic stroke and, especially for DBS surgery, device-related infection.[47,48] In large surgical series, the risk of symptomatic hemorrhage complicating DBS lead insertion is 1.5–3.0% per lead implant. The risk of a hemorrhage resulting in permanently increased morbidity is 0.5–1.0% per lead. This risk is increased in the setting of untreated hypertension, coagulopathy, or evidence on MRI of significant small vessel ischemic disease or extensive cerebral atrophy. Most clinicians require that a preoperative screening MRI of the brain be obtained, if not recently accomplished already, prior to making a final determination about surgical candidacy. The risk of serious infection of a newly implanted device, defined as an infection requiring reoperation to remove all or part of the implanted hardware, is 2–5% per device. Conditions that increase this risk, such as long-standing severe diabetes or need for chronic immunosuppression, are relative contraindications for device implantation. Such patients may be more appropriate candidates for unilateral pallidotomy.

Type of DBS neurostimulator

There are several commercially available DBS neurostimulators, each with different physical specifications and features. Determining which device to implant is based on patient diagnosis, body weight, device attributes, the need for unilateral or bilateral stimulation, and other factors. Availability of rechargeable neurostimulators will require additional candidate screening. Key factors in determining if a patient is a candidate for a rechargeable device are listed in Table 2.11.

Patient expectations and social support

Candidates for DBS should demonstrate a clear understanding of the procedures entailed in their treatment, potential risks of surgery, and realistic expectations about what can be achieved with DBS. Patients need to understand that DBS will not "cure" their disease or likely alter disease progression, and that the goal of DBS is suppression of motor symptoms and optimization of motor function and quality of life. Patients need to understand that the benefits of DBS will take time to accrue, since a number of visits may be required to optimize stimulator settings and the concomitant medication regimen. Patients and their families should be committed to working closely with the medical team in the postoperative management of their DBS therapy, both in the early postoperative period and over time.

Interdisciplinary and multidisciplinary consensus

An effective method for arriving at decisions regarding the candidacy of patients for treatment with DBS is to collect the required data for each patient and then convene a conference in which these details are discussed by the interdisciplinary/multidisciplinary team. This team is typically comprised of neurologists, neurosurgeons, nurses, neuropsychologists, and others who work together to evaluate and educate patients and their families. It is extremely useful to review together the medical history, motor testing scores, neurocognitive and psychiatric data, neuroimaging findings, and general clinical impressions. This process allows a consensus decision to be reached on the suitability of each particular patient for DBS treatment and fosters a consistent and cohesive treatment approach.

The determination of movement disorder patient candidacy for DBS surgery is still evolving. As surgical techniques advance and DBS hardware improves, the risk associated with this surgery will likely decrease. This may lead some physicians and patients to consider DBS surgery earlier in the course of the disease in the future. However, at this time, DBS is indicated for patients having a clear movement disorder diagnosis known to improve with DBS who are experiencing meaningful impairment from their symptoms, despite pharmacological management, in whom the potential risk associated with undergoing the implant surgery is deemed to be acceptable.

References

1. Weaver F, Follett K, Hur K, Ippolito D, Stern M. Deep brain stimulation in Parkinson disease: a metaanalysis of patient outcomes. *J Neurosurg* 2005;**103**:956–67.

2. Deuschl G, Schade-Brittinger C, Krack P, et al. A randomized trial of deep-brain stimulation for Parkinson's disease. *N Engl J Med* 2006;**355**:896–908.

3. Goetz CG. Rating scale for dyskinesia in Parkinson's disease. *Mov Disord* 1999;**14**:48–53.

4. Jenkinson C, Fitzpatrick R, Peto V. *The Parkinson's Disease Questionnaire. User Manual for the PDQ-39, PDQ-8, and PDQ Summary Index.* Oxford: Health Services Research Unit; 1998.

5. Charles PD, Van Blercom N, Krack P, et al. Predictors of effective bilateral subthalamic nucleus stimulation for PD. *Neurology* 2002;**59**:932–4.

6. Fahn S, Elton RL. Members of the UPDRS development committee. United Parkinson's Disease Rating Scale. In Fahn S, Marsden CD, Calne CB, Goldstien M, eds. *Recent Developments in Parkinson's Disease.* Florham Park, NJ: MacMillan Healthcare Information; 1987:153–63.

7. Pollak P. Deep brain stimulation. Annual Course of the American Academy of Neurology 2000. San Diego, CA; 2000.

8. Defer GL, Widner H, Marie RM, Remy P, Levivier M. Core assessment program for surgical interventional therapies in Parkinson's disease (CAPSIT-PD). *Mov Disord* 1999;**14**:572–84.

9. Aarsland D, Andersen K, Larsen JP, Lolk A, Kragh-Sorensen P. Prevalence and characteristics of dementia in Parkinson disease: an 8-year prospective study. *Arch Neurol* 2003;**60**:387–92.

10. Saint-Cyr JA, Trepanier LL, Kumar R, Lozano AM, Lang AE. Neuropsychological consequences of chronic bilateral stimulation of the subthalamic nucleus in Parkinson's disease. *Brain* 2000;**123**:2091–108.

11. Trepanier LL, Saint-Cyr JA, Lozano AM, Lang AE. Neuropsychological consequences of posteroventral pallidotomy for the treatment of Parkinson's disease. *Neurology* 1998;**51**:207–15.

12. Scott R, Gregory R, Hines N, et al. Neuropsychological, neurological and functional outcome following pallidotomy for Parkinson's disease. A consecutive series of eight simultaneous bilateral and twelve unilateral procedures. *Brain* 1998;**121**:659–75.

13. Zadikoff C, Fox SH, Tang-Wai DF, et al. A comparison of the mini mental state exam to the Montreal cognitive assessment in identifying cognitive deficits in Parkinson's disease. *Mov Disord* 2008;**23**:297–9.

14. The Montreal Cognitive Assessment (MoCA). http://www.mocatest.org. Accessed October 27, 2008.

15. Weintraub D, Stern MB. Psychiatric complications in Parkinson disease. *Am J Geriatr Psychiatry* 2005;**13**:844–51.

16. Troster A, Fields J, Wilkinson S, et al. Effect of motor improvement on quality of life following subthalamic stimulation is mediated by changes in depressive symptomatology. *Stereotact Funct Neurosurg* 2003;**80**:43–7.

17. Funkiewiez A, Ardouin C, Caputo E, et al. Long term effects of bilateral subthalamic nucleus stimulation on cognitive function, mood, and behaviour in Parkinson's disease. *J Neurol Neurosurg Psychiatry* 2004;**75**:834–9.

18. Saint-Cyr JA, Trepanier LL. Neuropsychologic assessment of patients for movement disorder surgery. *Mov Disord* 2000;**15**:771–83.

19. Doshi P, Chhaya N, Bhatt M. Depression leading to attempted suicide after bilateral subthalamic nucleus stimulation for Parkinson's disease. *Mov Disord* 2002;**17**:1084–5.

20. Sheikhi J, Yesavage J. Geriatric Depression Scale (GDS): recent evidence and development of a shorter version. In Brink TL, ed. *Clinical Gerontology: A Guide to Assessment and Intervention*. New York: Haworth Press; 1986:165–73.

21. Miyasaki JM, Shannon K, Voon V, et al. Practice parameter: evaluation and treatment of depression, psychosis, and dementia in Parkinson disease (an evidence-based review): report of the Quality Standards Subcommittee of the American Academy of Neurology. *Neurology* 2006;**66**:996–1002.

22. Lang AE, Widner H. Deep brain stimulation for Parkinson's disease: patient selection and evaluation. *Mov Disord* 2002;**17**(Suppl 3):S94–101.

23. Welter M, Houeto J, Tezenas du Montcel S, et al. Clinical predictive factors of subthalamic stimulation in Parkinson's disease. *Brain* 2002;**125**:575–83.

24. Tavella A, Bergamasco B, Bosticco E, et al. Deep brain stimulation of the subthalamic nucleus in Parkinson's disease: long-term follow-up. *Neurol Sci* 2002;**23** (Suppl 2):S111–12.

25. Ostrem J, Christine C, Starr P, Heath S, Marks W. Effect on patient age on response to subthalamic nucleus or globus pallidus deep brain stimulation for Parkinson's disease: results from a prospective, randomized study. *Neurology* 2004;**62**(Suppl 5):A396.

26. Kleiner-Fisman G, Fisman DN, et al. Long-term follow up of bilateral deep brain stimulation of the subthalamic nucleus in patients with advanced Parkinson disease. *J Neurosurg* 2003;**99**:489–95.

27. Mogilner AY, Sterio D, Rezai AR, et al. Subthalamic nucleus stimulation in patients with a prior pallidotomy. *J Neurosurg* 2002;**96**:660–5.

28. Weaver FM, Follett K, Hur K, Ippolito D, Stern M. Deep brain stimulation in Parkinson disease: a metaanalysis of patient outcomes. *J Neurosurg* 2005;**103**:956–67.

29. Follett KA, Weaver FM, Stern M, et al. for the CSP 468 Study Group. Pallidal versus subthalamic deep-brain stimulation for Parkinson's disease. *N Engl J Med* 2010;**362**:2077–91.

30. Follett KA. Comparision of pallidal and subthalamic deep brain stimulation for the treatment of levodopa-induced dyskinesias. *Neurosurg Focus* 2004;**17**(1):14–9.

31. Burchiel KJ, Anderson VC, Favre J, Hammerstad JP. Comparison of pallidal and subthalamic nucleus deep brain stimulation for advanced Parkinson's disease: results of a randomized, blinded pilot study. *Neurosurgery* 1999;**45**:1375–82; discussion 1382–4.

32. Vitek J. Deep brain stimulation for Parkinsons' disease. A critical re-evaluation of STN versus GPi DBS. *Stereotact Funct Neurosurg* 2002;**78**:119–31.

33. Putzke J, Wharen RJ, Wszolek Z, et al. Thalamic deep brain stimulation for tremor-predominant Parkinson's disease. *Parkinsonism Relat Disord* 2003;**10**(2):81–8.

34. Kumar R, Lozano AM, Sime E, Lang AE. Long-term follow-up of thalamic deep brain stimulation for essential and parkinsonian tremor. *Neurology* 2003;**61**:1601–4.

35. Jain S, Lo SE, Louis ED. Common misdiagnosis of a common neurological disorder: how are we misdiagnosing essential tremor? *Arch Neurol* 2006;**63**:1100–4.

36. Jankovic J. Essential tremor: a heterogeneous disorder. *Mov Disord* 2002;**17**:638–44.

37. Benito-Leon J, Louis ED. Clinical update: diagnosis and treatment of essential tremor. *Lancet* 2007;**369**:1152–4.

38. Zesiewicz TA, Elble R, Louis ED, et al. Practice parameter: therapies for essential tremor: report of the Quality Standards Subcommittee of the American Academy of Neurology. *Neurology* 2005;**64**:2008–20.

39. Findley LJ, Cleeves L, Calzetti S. Primidone in essential tremor of the hands and head: a double blind controlled clinical study. *J Neurol Neurosurg Psychiatry* 1985;**48**:911–5.

40. Ostrem JL, Starr PA. Treatment of dystonia with deep brain stimulation. *Neurotherapeutics* 2008;**5**:320–30.

41. Damier P, Thobois S, Witjas T, et al. Bilateral deep brain stimulation of the globus pallidus to treat tardive dyskinesia. *Arch Gen Psychiatry* 2007;**64**:170–6.

42. Comella CL, Leurgans S, Wuu J, Stebbins GT, Chmura T. Rating scales for dystonia: a multicenter assessment. *Mov Disord* 2003;**18**:303–12.

43. Burke RE, Fahn S, Marsden CD, et al. Validity and reliability of a rating scale for the primary torsion dystonias. *Neurology* 1985;**35**:73–7.

44. Comella CL, Stebbins GT, Goetz CG, et al. Teaching tape for the motor section of the Toronto Western Spasmodic Torticollis Scale. *Mov Disord* 1997;**12**:570–5.

45. Isaias IU, Alterman RL, Tagliati M. Outcome predictors of pallidal stimulation in patients with primary dystonia: the role of disease duration. *Brain* 2008;**131**:1895–902.

46. Starr PA, Turner RS, Rau G, et al. Microelectrode-guided implantation of deep brain stimulators into the globus pallidus internus for dystonia: techniques, electrode locations, and outcomes. *J Neurosurg* 2006;**104**:488–501.

47. Hariz MI. Complications of deep brain stimulation surgery. *Mov Disord* 2002;**17**(Suppl 3):S162–6.

48. Umemura A, Jaggi JL, Hurtig HI, et al. Deep brain stimulation for movement disorders: morbidity and mortality in 109 patients. *J Neurosurg* 2003;**98**:779–84.

49. Gelb DJ, Oliver E, Gilman S. Diagnostic criteria for Parkinson's disease. *Arch Neurol* 1999;**56**:33–9.

50. Bain P, Brin M, Deuschl G, et al. Criteria for the diagnosis of essential tremor. *Neurology* 2000;**54**:S7.

51. Deuschl G, Bain P, Brin M. Consensus statement of the Movement Disorder Society on Tremor Ad Hoc Scientific Committee. *Mov Disord* 1998;**13**(Suppl 3):2–23.

Chapter 3

Surgical placement of deep brain stimulation leads for the treatment of movement disorders: intraoperative aspects

Physiological mapping, test stimulation, and patient evaluation

Helen Bronte-Stewart

Introduction

Deep brain stimulation (DBS) for movement disorders consists of chronic high frequency electrical stimulation of certain targets in the basal ganglia, the deep gray matter of the brain. The success of the therapy relies on three main factors: the appropriate selection of patients, the accurate placement of the DBS lead in the sensorimotor regions of the target nuclei, and optimal choice of electrical parameters for stimulation. This chapter will focus on the second critical factor for success of DBS, namely the placement of the DBS lead. An increasing number of neurologists, physiologists, nurses, and others are being trained to be in the operating room to assist the neurosurgeon, and they serve an important role in optimizing DBS surgery.

Background

Basal ganglia anatomy – parallel distributed functional anatomy – allows for local therapy such as DBS

The basal ganglia are the deep nuclei of the brain (Figure 3.1). The input nuclei of the basal ganglia, the caudate, and putamen, receive excitatory input from almost all cortical areas and together make up the striatum. The main output nuclei are the internal segment of the globus pallidus (GPi) and the substantia nigra pars reticularis (SNpr). Sensorimotor information flows from the input nucleus (putamen) to the output nuclei (GPi and SNpr) through anatomically and neurochemically distinct projections, which may function as a "center-surround" mechanism to select the desired movement and inhibit unwanted movements. The GPi sends inhibitory outputs to pallidal receiving areas of the motor thalamus and brainstem nuclei. The nigrostriatal (dopaminergic) pathway from the substantia nigra pars compacta (SNpc) to the putamen acts to facilitate that process (Figure 3.1).

The subthalamic nucleus (STN) is an important nucleus in the functional organization of the basal ganglia.[1,2] The STN receives excitatory inputs from motor and premotor cortex and exerts a powerful excitatory effect on its target nuclei, GPi, globus pallidus externa (GPe), SNpr, SNpc, and the pedunculopontine nucleus (PPN).[1,3–6] Through fast conducting pathways, it is hypothesized the STN relays the overall cortical command (template) over the pallida, upon which the focusing of movement takes place through the slower, integrated striato-pallidal pathways. Information processing through the basal ganglia is believed to occur through functionally distinct circuits that are components of a network connecting cortical and subcortical structures. The circuits carrying sensorimotor versus oculomotor versus cognitive and associative information are largely segregated in different regions of each nucleus. Within the sensorimotor regions of each nucleus, there is somatotopic segregation of arm versus leg versus facial representation.

Deep Brain Stimulation Management, ed. William J. Marks, Jr. Published by Cambridge University Press.
© Cambridge University Press 2011.

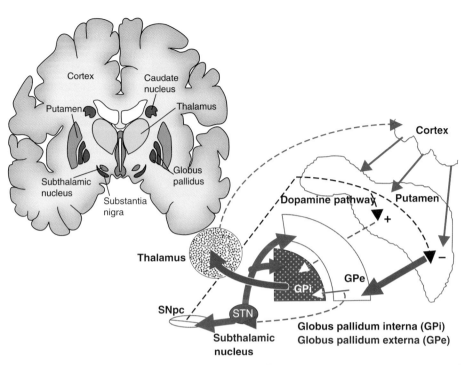

Figure 3.1 Schematic diagram of the nuclei and pathways of the basal ganglia. The nigrostriatal pathway from the substantia nigra pars compacta (SNpc) to the striatum is dopaminergic. In Parkinson's disease (PD), the results of dopamine deficiency include increased neuronal activity in the subthalamic nucleus (STN) and globus pallidus internus (GPi), with irregular and bursting neuronal firing patterns. Increased synchrony is found among sensorimotor networks, which may contribute to PD motor signs.

Movement disorders may be thought of as "brain arrhythmias": DBS as a brain pacemaker

Loss of dopaminergic input to the striatum results in the appearance of the classical motor signs of Parkinson's disease (PD). Dopamine depletion in the striatum results in an increase in neuronal activity in GPi and STN, which in turn leads to over-inhibition of thalamocortical and brainstem projections from the GPi. Mean neuronal firing rates are increased in both STN and GPi in MPTP-treated primates[2,3,7–10] and in patients with PD.[11,12] Experimental results in MPTP monkeys have shown that increased firing rates in both GPi and STN occur prior to the onset of symptoms.[13] Neuronal firing patterns in untreated PD are irregular, with oscillatory and bursting firing modes. In dystonia, firing patterns are also irregular and bursting but with lower mean firing rates. In tremor, firing patterns in basal ganglia nuclei and the thalamus are oscillatory and may be directly or indirectly correlated to the tremor frequency.[14]

A current theory is that the DBS system acts as a brain pacemaker. Chronic high frequency electrical stimulation of the target nucleus probably entrains irregular neuronal firing patterns and desynchronizes pathological hypersynchronization within sensorimotor circuits.[15,16]

DBS lead implantation

The goal is to place the DBS lead accurately in the center of the sensorimotor region of the target nucleus and/or in proximity to sensorimotor circuits traversing the region. Equally important is to avoid being close to other neighboring nuclei or fiber tracts, stimulation of which will cause adverse effects.

It is to be emphasized that DBS can be termed local therapy. Deep brain stimulation affects only local circuits and brain regions, unlike medication, which affects the whole body by transmission through the bloodstream. The effect of the electrical field produced by DBS falls off with the square of the distance from the electrical source.[17] Thus, accurate placement of the DBS lead in sensorimotor regions is critical to the success of the therapy.

DBS implantation is a team-based neurosurgical procedure, led by a neurosurgeon who should be trained in functional, stereotactic neurosurgery.

> The components of the DBS lead implant procedure typically include initial imaging-guided anatomical targeting, burr hole placement and headstage attachment, intraoperative microelectrode recording (MER), intraoperative micro-stimulation, and intraoperative macro-stimulation through the DBS lead after the DBS lead has been placed.

The members of the team working with the neurosurgeon are usually a neurologist and/or a neurophysiologist, an anesthesiologist, and other support personnel. The goal is to assist the neurosurgeon with the MER and to perform neurological testing of the patient during intraoperative micro-stimulation and DBS lead test stimulation. The procedure is usually performed with the patient awake and under local anesthesia only to allow this testing.

Anatomical targeting

> Precise anatomical targeting requires stereotactic functional techniques to identify the nucleus of interest and to calculate the first microelectrode trajectory, such that it traverses the sensorimotor region and avoids major cortical and subcortical blood vessels. Accurate targeting is the most important aspect of the procedure, upon which the other tasks rely.

If the first microelectrode pass is not even in the nucleus of choice, then finding the sensorimotor region within the nucleus is much harder and will require more MER passes to find the target.

A wide range of targeting techniques is currently used. In a recent survey of 36 North American DBS centers,[18] most sites used the stereotactic frame (Leksell, CRW, or Compass) for initial targeting and intraoperative electrode guidance, but a few used the frameless stereotactic technique. The frame-based and frameless techniques require preoperative imaging using MRI and/or MRI/CT fusion techniques for initial anatomical targeting. The frame-based

targeting uses fiducial markers on the frame as a guide, and thus the targeting is performed on the day of surgery. The frameless system is an image-guided system that uses fiducial markers on the skull and thus can be performed the day before surgery.[19] A comparison study has shown that the accuracy of DBS lead placement was not significantly different between the frame-based and frameless systems.[19] Both had an error margin of 3.5 mm from the expected target to the actual location of the lead. This may be significant in these small, deep structures since a small deviation from the planned target could place the stimulating lead outside the nucleus (for example, close to the internal capsule) and/or in a cognitive or associative region within the nucleus. Current potential imaging and surgical errors include a 2–3 mm error in MRI targeting, errors in MRI/CT fusion techniques, the potential of brain shift when replacing the mapping electrode with the DBS lead (see below), and the potential brain shift that may occur over time in the operating room due to CSF loss.

Intraoperative microelectrode recording (MER)

Studies from ablative procedures such as pallidotomy and from DBS procedures have confirmed that the optimal location of the lesion or DBS lead spans the sensorimotor region of the target nucleus.[12,20–24] The sensorimotor regions of the basal ganglia nuclei are anatomically segregated in terms of somatotopy and function and may have quite irregular shapes (Figure 3.2). Sensorimotor circuits mediating simple motor actions are situated in the dorsolateral aspect of the STN, whereas associative and cognitive function appears to be situated in the medial pole of the STN (Figure 3.2a).[25,26] Due to the small size of the STN, deviations from the sensorimotor region of the nucleus to the medial portion of the nucleus risk affecting associative STN and potentially causing stimulation-induced cognitive or psychiatric side effects. The distance between these regions can be as small as 3–4 mm and so it is especially important to try to place the DBS lead in the center of the sensorimotor region.

> MER allows precise identification of the sensorimotor region in each nucleus and compensates for any anatomical targeting errors.

(a)

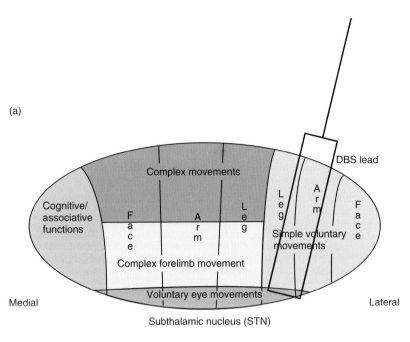

DBS lead

Complex movements

Cognitive/
associative
functions

F
a
c
e

A
r
m

L
e
g

L
e
g

A
r
m

F
a
c
e

Simple voluntary
movements

Complex forelimb movement

Voluntary eye movements

Medial

Lateral

Subthalamic nucleus (STN)

(b)

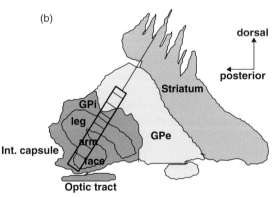

dorsal

posterior

Striatum

GPi

leg

arm

GPe

Int. capsule

face

Optic tract

Figure 3.2 The anatomical segregation of function and somatotopy in the subthalamic nucleus (STN) (a) and globus pallidus internus (GPi) (b). Within the STN there is anatomical segregation of simple versus complex movement, eye movement, mood, and cognitive function. The proper position of the deep brain stimulation lead is represented in each nucleus.

MER techniques vary from institution to institution regarding the use of single neuronal (high impedance, microelectrode) versus multi-unit (lower impedance, semi-microelectrode) recording and whether one or several microelectrode passes are made to determine the final location for the DBS lead. The North American survey revealed that all centers used some form of intraoperative electrical confirmation of the DBS lead placement, and over 95% used electrophysiological recording.[18] Most centers use multi-pass MER to identify the sensorimotor region, with an average of 2.3 ± 1.4 passes per case. Several studies have shown that the use of MER in addition to anatomical targeting proved to be more precise than surgical targeting based solely on anatomical information provided by a T2-weighted MRI.[27–29] However, concern has been expressed that using multiple microelectrode passes to define and map the target structure could increase morbidity and add risk to the patient.[30] One large multicenter trial of DBS for PD (268 cases) suggested that microelectrode recording may increase the risk of hemorrhage,[31] but this was not found to be a significant cause of hemorrhage in another large single center study of DBS in 481 cases.[32] In our experience, intraoperative MER does not cause morbidity and improves bradykinesia even before placement of the DBS lead.[33]

MER: method for determining anatomical boundaries and the sensorimotor region

A 0.5–1.0 megOhm platinum–iridium microelectrode is inserted into a guide tube (or cannula) lined with Teflon to reduce microphonics. The entire microelectrode/guide tube assembly is carried by a motorized micro-drive mounted on a head stage. The microelectrode is advanced within its guide tube to a depth of 15 mm above the target. It is then slowly advanced beyond the guide tube as the MER takes place to and below the target depth at the nucleus. A scribe notates the activity encountered and the depth of each

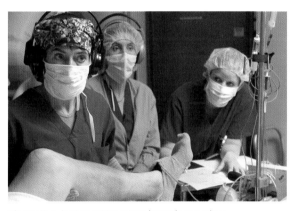

Figure 3.3 Intraoperative microelectrode recording. The neurologist or neurophysiologist listens to and watches on an oscilloscope the response of neurons as she rapidly and repetitively moves each joint about its axis on the contralateral side of the body. A scribe notes all the responses.

encounter, which provides a "route map" for each MER track. The neurologist or neurophysiologist stands alongside the patient, not in the sterile field (Figure 3.3). In most cases both the neurosurgeon and neurologist/neurophysiologist are wearing headphones. The brain's electrical activity is amplified from the deep recording electrode and fed through the headphones and displayed on an oscilloscope. The patient is awake and needs to be able to cooperate with the neurologist and neurosurgeon.

Mapping the sensorimotor region

The first microelectrode track follows the initial trajectory determined by the stereotactic planning. Some centers use a cylinder with five microelectrodes in a concentric array, from which multiple recordings are made during one pass. Other centers use multipass MER, using a single microelectrode, where subsequent tracks are made depending on the electrophysiological findings obtained during the previous track. Single neuronal unit or multi-unit recordings may be obtained. Each unit or group of units is tested for responses to both contralateral arm and leg passive and/or active movement. Within the upper extremity, responses are tested for movement about the metacarpophalangeal, wrist, elbow, and shoulder joints. Within the lower extremity, responses are tested for movement about the ankle, knee, and hip joints. A movement is made about each joint in the flexion and extension directions separately, rather than in a smooth "sinusoidal" motion. Figure 3.4

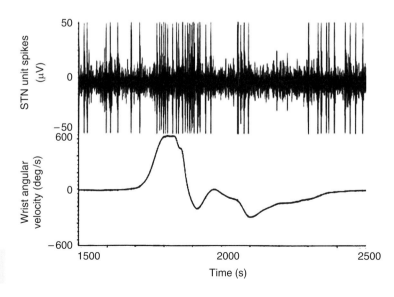

Figure 3.4 Microelectrode recording consists of recording the response of neurons to passive and active movement. A subthalamic nucleus unit has an irregular, baseline firing pattern and shows an increase in firing rate as the wrist is passively extended. Angular velocity was measured using a solid-state gyroscope attached to the dorsum of the hand. Reproduced with permission from *Journal of Neurosurgery*, April, 2004, **100**, 4, Microelectrode recording revealing a somatotopic body map in the subthalamic nucleus in humans with Parkinson disease, Romanelli, 611–18.

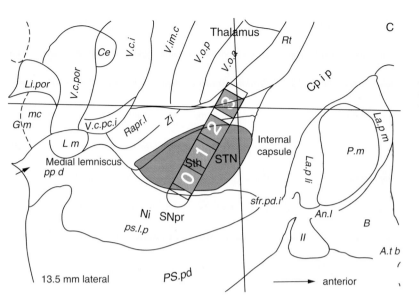

Figure 3.5 A sagittal section of the subthalamic nucleus adapted from the Schaltenbrand–Bailey atlas, on which has been placed the position of a deep brain stimulation lead (Medtronic model 3389) as determined from the angle of entry and microelectrode recording mapping of the sensorimotor region.

shows the increase in firing rate of a neuron that is clearly responding to sensorimotor input, rapid wrist extension movement.

Boundary and sensorimotor mapping using MER

Microelectrode recording determines accurately the dorsal and ventral borders of the target nuclei and the sensorimotor regions within. Each nucleus trajectory has a distinctive physiological "signature" and will be described briefly separately.

1. **STN** – the MER track usually passes through thalamus before entering STN (Figure 3.5). If the pass is anterior there is little neuronal activity in thalamus as the track passes through the reticular nuclei. The more posterior the pass the more "active" is the spontaneous activity in the thalamus as the microelectrode passes through the ventrolateral nuclei (Voa, Vop, Vim). In these nuclei the electrode may pick up the distinctive activity of "bursters," units with intermittent bursts of action potentials and an otherwise quiet baseline. As the electrode passes through the base of the thalamus, there is a clear drop in electrical activity as it enters white matter. This silence lasts until the dorsal border of STN is reached, except for the occasional cell that reflects passage through the zona incerta (Zi) (Figure 3.5). The dorsal border of STN is very clear, as there

is a dramatic increase in background spontaneous electrical activity. Neuronal activity is irregular and may be oscillatory or bursting in nature. As soon as a single cell or group of cells is isolated, the team begins to map for sensorimotor responses as detailed above. Usually the most dense neuronal activity and sensorimotor "driving" are in the dorsal aspects of the track. At the base of STN there is usually a distinct drop in background activity. The ventral border of STN is followed by entry into SNpr, which is quite distinct electrophysiologically, due to the regularity of firing patterns of SNpr neurons. If there is no gap or less than a 1 mm gap between STN and SNpr, this is a good guide that the MER location is central in the anterior–posterior plane and one indicator of a good position, given that there was sensorimotor driving within that pass.

2. **GPi** – the microelectrode track passes through striatum, GPe, and then GPi (Figure 3.6, Figure 3.2b). Each nucleus has distinct electrophysiological features. As the microelectrode passes through the striatum, spontaneous unit firing is evident, which is phasic (that is, it decreases to silence after a few seconds if the microelectrode remains stationary). New units are activated as the electrode advances. As the electrode moves from striatum to GPe there may be a lamina of white matter, which is silent (Figure 3.6). The entrance to GPe is noted by

25

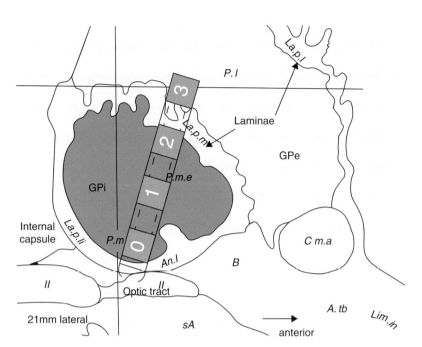

Figure 3.6 A sagittal section of the pallidum adapted from the Schaltenbrand–Bailey atlas, on which has been placed the position of a deep brain stimulation lead (Medtronic model 3387) as determined from the angle of entry and microelectrode recording mapping of the sensorimotor region.

activation of units with a more tonic pattern (that is, they persist if the electrode remains in that spot). The background activity remains low, so that GPe activity can be difficult to distinguish from that in striatum. Two distinct types of neuronal patterns are found in GPe, the high frequency pausing cells (pausers) and low frequency bursting cells (bursters). The pausers may be difficult to distinguish from striatal units, but as stated above, their firing will persist and with experience these are quite easy to identify. The bursters are very easy to identify, as they fire at low frequencies with bursts of high frequency spikes. These are signature units for GPe. As the electrode advances from GPe to GPi there is usually almost 1 mm of silence, reflecting passage through another lamina. The entrance to GPi in PD is characteristic for a dramatic increase in background activity with high frequency (70–90 Hz) discharging units. Sensorimotor mapping, as detailed above, commences with entry into GPi. As the microelectrode exits GPi, recording continues while the neurologist/neurophysiologist shines a light into the patient's eyes, to activate fibers of the optic tract. If the optic tract lies immediately deep to GPi this is a good sign of placement.

3. **Vim-thalamus** – the goal is to place the DBS lead in the Vim/Vop nuclei of the ventral thalamus for tremor. In the thalamus the easiest way to determine the best location for the DBS lead with MER is to identify first the sensory nucleus (Vc), which forms the posterior border of Vim and is easily identified, as the cells respond to light tactile input such as brushing of the skin. Units that have deep kinesthetic responses characterize the border of Vc and Vim; they respond (increase their firing rate) to muscle squeezing and/or tendon tapping. The "kinesthetic" units in Vim respond to classic sensorimotor input (moving of the limbs) as seen in STN and GPi. The other electrophysiological firing pattern that helps to guide placement is the oscillatory firing pattern of units in Vop and Vim, which may or may not be firing at similar frequencies to that of the limb tremor. The mediolateral plane determines the appropriate somatotopic location. The ventrolateral thalamus has an "onion-skin" pattern of somatotopy, where from lateral to medial directions are leg, arm, and face representations. If the patient has significant arm and chin tremor, for instance, the DBS lead should be targeted slightly more medial than if the patient has arm and leg tremor. In our center,

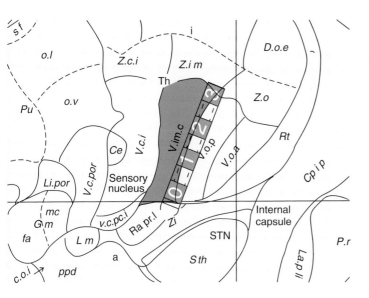

Figure 3.7 A sagittal section of the thalamus adapted from the Schaltenbrand–Bailey atlas, on which has been placed the position of a deep brain stimulation lead (Medtronic model 3387) as determined from the angle of entry and microelectrode recording mapping.

anatomical targeting aims for the implant track to be in Vim/Vop, with the target base at the base of the thalamus, at the appropriate mediolateral coordinate. However, the first MER track is then performed 3 mm posterior to that in order to identify Vc and the posterior border of Vim. If this is accomplished, the second track is performed 3 mm anterior to the first.

Micro-stimulation at the base of every MER track

At the base of each MER track micro-stimulation is performed to test for adverse effects; when present, these suggest close proximity of the MER track to surrounding neural structures intended to be avoided (such as the internal capsule). Micro-stimulation may also show beneficial results, such as reduction in tremor. Micro-stimulation is done through the cannula (guide tube) surrounding the microelectrode, so that the tip of the electrode is not damaged by stimulation. Cannula stimulation consists of trains of high frequency (~200 Hz) stimulation with currents from 0.5 to 5.0 milliamps (mA). Proximity to the internal capsule is determined, for all nuclei, by whether there is any noticeable twitching or contraction of muscles coincident with stimulation. It is important to monitor for facial muscle and/or palate or tongue movement, as these motor fibers pass through the capsule at similar coordinates to the sensorimotor regions of the target nuclei. A common and not necessarily problematic

effect elicited by micro-stimulation is the sensation of paresthesia. These usually are transient and resolve over 5–10 seconds. If they persist and/or occur at very low currents, though, then the MER track in STN or thalamus may be too posterior (Figures 3.5 and 3.7). Micro-stimulation at the base of GPi should always include testing of stimulation of the optic tract (Figure 3.6). The patient is asked to close their eyes, the room lights are usually dimmed, and the patient is asked to report whether they see any positive visual phenomena ("phosphenes") with stimulation. For all nuclei it is important to also check speech, as the current intensity is increased to determine whether dysarthria is being induced. The threshold at which side effects and/or beneficial responses occur is noted.

DBS lead insertion and intraoperative DBS test stimulation

Following removal of the microelectrode and cannula, the DBS lead is threaded into its guide tube and carefully driven to the target depth along the desired track or at the desired coordinates. Once the DBS lead has been placed at the target depth, intraoperative macro-stimulation using the DBS lead is performed to test for optimal placement. The neurosurgeon hands the end of the DBS lead from the sterile field to the neurologist or other assistant, who connects it to an external stimulator. The goal of intraoperative DBS test stimulation is to assess the efficacy of placement and the "therapeutic window" of stimulation.

Ideally a neurologist trained in movement disorders should perform this assessment.

The DBS lead is a linear tetrode: it has 4 cylindrical electrodes (diameter = 1.27 mm, length = 1.5 mm) with an inter-contact distance of 1.5 mm (model 3387, Medtronic, Inc.) or 0.5 mm (model 3389, Medtronic, Inc.). Stimulation may be through any one or several electrodes on the lead in a monopolar (unipolar) mode or through any pair of electrodes in a bipolar mode. Thus, stimulation through different electrodes or combinations of electrodes will result in a different topography of electrical field. Intraoperative DBS test stimulation may be done through a dipole across all the contacts (designating the most distal electrode, 0, as negative and the most proximal electrode, 3, as positive), but some clinicians may choose to assess the therapeutic window across each electrode in a monopolar fashion in the operating room. Variable parameters are electrode polarity, amplitude, pulse width, and rate. In general, intraoperative testing is conducted using parameters similar to those that will be typically used clinically for therapeutic purposes on a chronic basis to assess for benefit and for stimulation-induced adverse effects.

A useful rule is that with a properly located DBS lead in any of the target nuclei used to treat movement disorders, stimulation-induced adverse effects are not expected to occur at low-to-medium levels of stimulation. By virtue of the close proximity of neighboring neural structures to the anatomical target of therapeutic stimulation, though, stimulation-induced adverse effects are expected to occur (and should be seen) at medium-to-high levels of stimulation.

In PD and tremor disorders, there should be immediate relief of some of the patient's signs and symptoms with intraoperative DBS test stimulation. If there is no efficacy at even high amplitudes of stimulation, then this suggests that the placement of the DBS lead is not optimal or that there is a technical problem preventing the stimulating current from reaching the brain. If there is some efficacy but stimulation-related side effects occur at low amplitudes then this suggests that the DBS lead is in or near the sensorimotor region but not optimally placed in the center of the region. There may not be any difference in symptoms in patients with dystonia, though, and then the goal is purely to test the amplitude threshold for adverse effects. A few

guidelines to placement of the DBS lead in each nucleus are given below.

Subthalamic nucleus (STN)

The base of the lead should not extend far into the SNpr due to possible adverse effects of depression with stimulation in SNpr. Intraoperative STN DBS test stimulation in PD requires assessment of motor improvement along with potential adverse effects as the amplitude is increased, such as changes in speech and/or motor function (indicating proximity to internal capsule, with the lead too anterior or lateral to the desired location), persistent paresthesia (indicating proximity to medial lemniscus, with the lead too posterior to the desired location), eye deviation (indicating that the lead is too medial and deep to the desired location), mood or cognitive changes (indicating that the lead is too medial to the desired location), or eyelid opening apraxia (indicating that the lead is possibly dorsal or associated with the oculomotor loop through STN). With intraoperative test stimulation of the DBS lead in the STN the patient may acutely develop dyskinesia. This is usually a sign of a well-placed DBS lead but is not a necessary feature. The efficacy of the placement may be detected by testing rigidity and tremor. However, these signs and symptoms may have resolved purely from the MER mapping process, due to a "micro-lesion" effect. We have employed quantitative measures of bradykinesia and have shown that these improve significantly in the STN in PD after MER alone and with intraoperative DBS test stimulation.[33] We use this measure to check for efficacy. Figure 3.8 shows the improvement in limb bradykinesia after MER alone and during intraoperative stimulation using the DBS lead.

Globus pallidus (GPi)

In PD it has been shown that differential stimulation in ventral and dorsal aspects of GPi result in different effects (Figure 3.6).[34,35] Ventral stimulation of GPi for PD improves rigidity and suppresses dyskinesia but has a limited effect on bradykinesia, whereas dorsal stimulation improves bradykinesia but can worsen dyskinesia, possibly due to overflow stimulation of GPe. Intraoperative GPi DBS test stimulation should assess improvement and adverse effects that occur, such as visual phenomena (indicating that the DBS lead is too deep if this effect occurs at relatively low amplitudes of stimulation) and changes in speech and/or motor function (indicating that the DBS lead is too posterior and/or medial if this effect occurs at relatively low amplitudes of stimulation). Careful

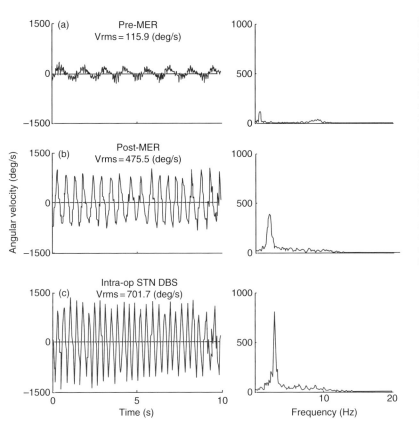

Figure 3.8 Angular velocity traces of repetitive wrist pronation–supination movements, from a subject with Parkinson's disease, off medication in the operating room, before any instrumentation of the brain (a), after microelectrode recording (MER) (b), and during intraoperative subthalamic nucleus deep brain stimulation (STN DBS) test stimulation (c). The MER alone resulted in improvement in upper extremity bradykinesia (b). Further improvement was seen during intraoperative stimulation using the DBS lead (c). Reproduced with permission from Movement Disorders, January, 2006, Improvement in a quantitative measure of bradykinesia after microelectrode recording in patients with Parkinson's disease during deep brain stimulation surgery. Miller et al. 673–8.

visual field testing should focus on the inferior quadrants, which is where a field defect is most likely to occur.

Vim thalamus

In the ventrolateral thalamus, the DBS lead is usually targeted to the Vim nucleus, at an angle that includes the posterior portion of Vop and places the lead 1–3 mm anterior to the border of the Vim and Vc (sensory) nuclei (Figure 3.7). The base of the DBS lead should be aligned with the base of the Vim nucleus, usually in the plane of the anterior and posterior commissures. Intraoperative DBS test stimulation should assess improvement in tremor and occurrence of adverse effects induced by relatively low amplitudes of stimulation of persistent paresthesia (indicating that the DBS lead is too posterior and stimulation is affecting the Vc), dysarthria (indicating that the DBS lead is too deep), or tonic muscle contractions (indicating that the DBS lead is too lateral, causing involvement of the internal capsule). For Vim DBS it is important not to place the lead too anterior, ideally only about

2 mm anterior to the border of Vc, to avoid side effects of stimulation of the internal capsule. Paresthesia noted in the operating room (stimulation volume reaching Vc) will often be transient and adapt over time. However, capsular side effects of muscle contraction will not and will limit the efficacy of DBS.

Once the DBS lead has been inserted and it has been verified that it is in the optimal location, the outer guide tube is carefully removed and the lead is secured to the skull, the rest of the lead is coiled, and the skin is closed.

Making the map

A map should be made of the position of the DBS lead in the nucleus of choice, as this will help the clinician who ultimately performs the programming of the DBS system, especially if the programmer was not in the operating room. One commonly employed method is to record the depth and type of each unit's response during MER on a scaled piece of graph paper and transfer this onto clear film. Passes in the same plane are transcribed onto the same film, and passes in different mediolateral planes are transcribed on separate films. An "x" marking the target depth of the first track is marked on each film. Absent responses are also recorded. The clear films are over-laid onto a custom-made set of scaled, translucent parasagittal planes from the Schaltenbrand–Bailey atlas, at the appropriate mediolateral coordinates, and the "x"s are aligned. The anterior–posterior entry angle of the tracks is calculated and laid under the translucent maps so that the tracks are oriented cor-rectly. This results in a three-dimensional map of the sensorimotor region and nuclear boundaries of the target nucleus on a rough outline of the target's anat omy. This constitutes the electrophysiological spatial map of optimal placement of the DBS lead. Figures 3.5, 3.6, and 3.7 show the maps of the placement of the DBS lead on appropriate planes of each target nucleus.

Postoperative imaging: lead location confirmation

It is important to obtain some imaging feedback of the site of placement of the DBS lead, either using intraoperative radiographs (if ventriculography is performed) or fluoroscopy, or postoperative CT or MRI (following the device manufacturer's safety guidelines) to confirm that the DBS lead placement is at the site intended and that it has not moved after securing it at the scalp. The North American survey revealed that postoperative imaging to confirm the site of DBS lead placement was performed by 92% of centers, most using MRI and fewer using CT or ventriculography.[18] The neurologist may assist in this and should always perform a postoperative assess-ment of the patient to check for any adverse effects after the final placement of the DBS lead.

Pitfalls and potential sources of error in the outcome of DBS lead placement

There are several reasons why a patient may not have a good outcome from DBS, including poor patient selection, co-morbidities, suboptimal DBS lead place-ment, and inadequate post-DBS programming. In a study of 41 patients who were referred to 2 DBS

centers for poor outcome from DBS at other centers, 19 (46%) were judged to have had improperly placed DBS leads, whereas 24% had inaccurate diagnoses.[36] Of the 19 misplaced leads, 7 were able to be replaced and provide the patient with symptom improve-ment. Poor placement can result from lack of use of intraoperative physiological mapping techniques ("anatomical" placement), use of purely macrostimu-lation-guided lead placement without the use of MER, misinterpretation of the MER map, failure to place the DBS lead in the intended location after removal of the MER device, brain shift during the procedure resulting in a mismatch of the actual site of the target compared to preoperative targeting, and inadequate stabilization of the DBS lead after final placement (leading to retraction of the lead from its intended site). Methods to eliminate any and all of these poten-tial sources of error will improve the outcomes of a substantial percentage of patients.

References

1. Feger J, Hassani O, Mouroux M. The subthalamic nucleus and its connections. New electrophysiological and pharmacological data. *Adv Neurol* 1997;**74**:31–43.
2. DeLong M. Primate models of movement disorders of basal ganglia origin. *Trends Neurosci* 1990;**13**:281–85.
3. Wichmann T, Bergman H, DeLong M. The primate subthalamic nucleus. I. Functional properties in intact animals. *J Neurophysiol* 1994;**72**(2):494–506.
4. Robledo P, Feger J. Excitatory influence of rat subthalamic nucleus to substantia nigra pars reticulata and the pallidal complex: electrophysiological data. *Brain Res* 1990;**51**(8):47–54.
5. Kita H, Kitai S. Intracellular study of rat globus pallidus neurons: membrane properties and responses to neostriatal, subthalamic and nigral stimulation. *Brain Res* 1991;**564**:296–305.
6. Hammond C, Deniau J, Rizk A, Feger J. Electrophysiological demonstration of an excitatory subthalamonigral pathway in the rat. *Brain Res* 1978;**151**:235–44.
7. Miller W, DeLong M. *Altered Tonic Activity of Neurons in the Globus Pallidus and Subthalamic Nucleus in the Primate MPTP Model of Parkinsonism.* New York: Plenum Press; 1987.
8. Filion M, Tremblay L. Abnormal spontaneous activity of globus pallidus neurons in monkeys with MPTP-induced parkinsonism. *Brain Res* 1991;**547**:142–51.
9. Bergman H, Wichmann T, Karmon B, DeLong M. The primate subthalamic nucleus. II. Neuronal activity in the MPTP model of parkinsonism. *J Neurophysiol* 1994;**72**:507–20.

10. Bergman H, Wichmann T, DeLong M. Reversal of experimental parkinsonism by lesions of the subthalamic nucleus. *Science* 1990;**249**:1436–8.

11. Lozano A, Hutchison W, Kiss Z, et al. Methods for microelectrode-guided posteroventral pallidotomy. *J Neurosurg* 1996;**84**:192–202.

12. Vitek J, Bakay R, Hashimoto T, et al. Microelectrode-guided pallidotomy: technical approach and its application in medically intractable Parkinson's disease. *J Neurosurg* 1998;**88**:1027–43.

13. Bezard E, Boraud T, Bioulae B, Gross C. Presymptomatic revelation of experimental parkinsonism. *Neuro Report* 1997;**8**:435–8.

14. Lenz FA, Tasker RR, Kwan HC, et al. Single unit analysis of the human ventral thalamic nuclear group: correlation of thalamic "tremor cells" with the 3–6 Hz component of parkinsonian tremor. *J Neurosci* 1988;**8**:754–64.

15. Brown P. Oscillatory nature of human basal ganglia activity: relationship to the pathophysiology of Parkinson's disease. *Mov Disord* 2003;**18**(4):357–63.

16. Bronte-Stewart H, Barberini C, Miller Koop M, et al. The STN beta band profile in Parkinson's disease is stationary and shows prolonged attenuation after deep brain stimulation. *Exp Neurol* 2009;**215**:20–8.

17. McIntyre CC, Grill WM, Sherman DL, et al. Cellular effects of deep brain stimulation: model-based analysis of activation and inhibition. *J Neurophysiol* 2004;**91**:1457–69.

18. Ondo W, Bronte-Stewart H. The North American Survey of Placement and Adjustment Strategies for Deep Brain Stimulation. *Stereotact Funct Neurosurg* 2005;**83**(4):142–7.

19. Holloway KL, Gaede SE, Starr PA, et al. Frameless stereotaxy using bone fiducial markers for deep brain stimulation. *J Neurosurg* 2005;**103**(3):404–13.

20. Svennilson E, Torvik A, Lowe R, Leksell L. Treatment of parkinsonism by stereotactic thermolesions in the pallidal region. *Acta Psychiatr Scand* 1960;**35**:358–77.

21. Vitek J, Bakay R, DeLong M. Microelectrode-guided pallidotomy for medically intractable Parkinson's disease. *Adv Neurol* 1997;**74**:183–98.

22. Gross R, Lombardi W, Lang A, et al. Relationship of lesion location to clinical outcome following microelectrode-guided pallidotomy for Parkinson's disease. *Brain* 1999;**122**:405–16.

23. Eskandar E, Cosgrove G, Shinobu L, Penney J. The importance of accurate lesion placement in posteroventral pallidotomy: report of two cases. *J Neurosurg* 1998;**89**:630–4.

24. Bronte-Stewart H, Hill B, Molander M, et al. Lesion location predicts clinical outcome of pallidotomy. *Mov Disord* 1998;**13**:300.

25. Romanelli P, Heit G, Hill B, et al. Microelectrode recording reveals somatotopic body map in parkinsonian subthalamic nucleus of humans. *J Neurosurg* 2004;**100**:611–18.

26. Romanelli P, Bronte-Stewart HM, Heit G, Schaal DW, Vincenzo E. The functional organization of the sensorimotor region of the subthalamic nucleus. *Stereotact Funct Neurosurg* 2004;**82**:222–9.

27. Starr PA, Vitek JL, DeLong M, Bakay RA. Magnetic resonance imaging-based stereotactic localization of the globus pallidus and subthalamic nucleus. *Neurosurgery* 1999;**44**(2):303–13.

28. Bejjani BP, Dormont D, Pidoux B, et al. Bilateral subthalamic stimulation for Parkinson's disease by using three-dimensional stereotactic magnetic resonance imaging and electrophysiological guidance. *J Neurosurg* 2000;**92**(4):615–25.

29. Cuny E, Grehl D, Burbaud P, et al. Lack of agreement between direct magnetic resonance imaging and statistical determination of a subthalamic target: the role of electrophysiological guidance. *J Neurosurg* 2002;**97**:591–7.

30. Okun MS, Vitek JL. Lesion therapy for Parkinson's disease and other movement disorders: update and controversies. *Mov Disord* 2004; **19**(4):375–89.

31. Deep Brain Stimulation for Parkinson's Disease Study Group. Deep brain stimulation of the subthalamic nucleus or the pars interna of the globus pallidus in Parkinson's disease. *N Engl J Med* 2001;**345**:956–63.

32. Binder DK, Rau GM, Starr PA. Risk factors for hemorrhage during microelectrode-guided deep brain stimulator implantation for movement disorders. *Neurosurgery* 2005;**6**(4):722–32.

33. Miller Koop M, Andrzejewski A, Hill BC, Heit G, Bronte-Stewart, HM. Improvement in a quantitative measure of bradykinesia after microelectrode recording in patients with Parkinson's disease during deep brain stimulation surgery. *Mov Disord* 2006;**21**(5):673–8.

34. Bejjani B, Damier P, Arnulf I, et al. Pallidal stimulation for Parkinson's disease. Two targets? *Neurology* 1997;**49**:1564–9.

35. Pollak P, Benabid AL, Krack P, et al. Deep brain stimulation. In Jankovic J, Tolosa E, eds. *Parkinson's Disease and Movement Disorders*. Baltimore: Williams and Wilkins; 1998:1085–101.

36. Okun MS, Tagliati M, Pourfar M, et al. Management of referred deep brain stimulation failures: a retrospective analysis from 2 movement disorders centers. *Arch Neurol* 2005; **62**(8):1250–5.

31

Principles of neurostimulation

Erwin B. Montgomery, Jr.

Introduction

This chapter serves to introduce electrophysiological and electrical principles that underlie deep brain stimulation (DBS), with the purpose of facilitating effective and efficient postoperative programming. Indeed, it will be argued that anyone who sets their goal as efficient and effective programming will best be served by utilizing these principles. Understanding the present limitations regarding the practical DBS programming knowledge argues for the use of these fundamental principles. Further, even as the field of DBS rapidly expands in terms of indications, targets, and methodologies, knowledge of these principles will well serve the clinician because these principles are fundamental to electrophysiologically based therapies.

Background

Early on in the evolution of DBS, it was thought that high frequency DBS inhibits the target structure because of the analogous clinical outcomes between ablative procedures and DBS, namely pallidotomy and DBS of the globus pallidus internus (GPi) segment and between thalamotomy and thalamic DBS. Conversely, worsening of some symptoms and signs in Parkinson's disease with low frequency DBS led to the extension that low frequency DBS excites the target. Thus, the presumption was that DBS in situations that previously responded to surgical ablation, which accounts for the majority of DBS applications, would require high frequency DBS.

There is clear evidence that both high and low frequency DBS excite the outputs of the stimulated target[1-3] as well as afferent axons to the stimulated target[3] and axons passing in the vicinity of the

stimulated target.[4] In non-human primates, the direct neuronal responses in multiple nuclei of the basal ganglia–thalamic–cortical system show the same qualitative response, although the responses vary in magnitude.[3] It also is clear that some symptoms in a variety of disorders respond better to low frequency compared to high frequency DBS.[5,6]

In order to comprehensively explore the effects of DBS, the entire set of electrode configurations and stimulation parameters would have to be systematically tested. Configurations refer to the combination of active electrodes, negative (cathode) or positive (anode), in the usual multi-electrode arrays in commercially available DBS leads. Parameters refer to the characteristics of the stimulation, such as amplitude, pulse width, and rate. It is impractical, though, to explore every possible combination of electrode and stimulator settings and the clinical responses for each pertinent symptom for every disease.

Consequently, one has to turn to an explicit understanding of the underlying principles relevant to the DBS mechanisms of action.

There are at least three perspectives with respect to mechanisms of action. The first is the effects of DBS on neural elements such as axons, axon terminals, dendrites, and cell bodies, particularly in the electrical activities generated. The second relates to how the electrical activities generated in the neural elements are propagated through the basal ganglia–thalamic–cortical system, the brain regions relevant to movement disorders. There is considerable evidence that the therapeutic efficacy of DBS is related to its effects on the entire basal ganglia–thalamic–cortical system.[3,4]A third and most common perspective is the effects of DBS on neurotransmitters[7] and other neuromodulators.[8] However, conceptually, changes in neurotransmitters and neuromodulators relate directly to the electrical effects of DBS on neural elements. In the case of neurotransmitters, the depolarization due to action potentials arriving at the axonal terminals at the synapse generates the release of neurotransmitters.

There is considerable evidence that DBS-related changes in neurotransmitters and neuromodulators are unlikely to fully explain the DBS mechanisms of action. The time course of neurotransmitter and neuromodulator release is too coarse relative to the time scale of the DBS effect. For example, therapeutic DBS at a rate of 130 pulses per second (pps) has an inter-stimulus interval of approximately 7 ms, while ineffective DBS at 100 pps has an inter-stimulus interval of 10 ms. Thus, the difference between an effective and ineffective DBS rate is on the order of 3 ms, which is much too fast to be accounted for solely by a neurotransmitter and neuromodulator time course of action. Further, the success of DBS in patients with Parkinson's disease in the face of failed symptom improvement from clear neurotransmitter replacement, such as fetal cell transplantation,[9] is a strong argument against this third perspective.

The second perspective of systems-wide effects of DBS is much more problematic. While there are a number of hypotheses how these systems-wide effects may be therapeutic,[3] any complete understanding is at a distance. There are two general schemas, first that the therapeutic effects are local to the DBS target and the second being that the therapeutic DBS effect is a systems effect. While the number and range of neuronal responses to DBS is increasingly understood, which of these is causal to DBS efficacy is unknown. The truth of the matter is that the true mechanisms are unknown. This means that principles related to the systems-wide effects are unavailable to guide postoperative DBS management, at least at the present time.

> Fortunately, there is considerable knowledge and understanding of the effects of DBS on the neural elements. The most common effects are excitation of action potentials in axons to, from, and passing by the structures targeted by the electrodes on the DBS lead. Consequently, an understanding of the electrophysiological properties of action potentials in axons can be exploited to assist in postoperative DBS management.

The purpose of this chapter is to explain those processes.

Rough approximation of effective DBS

In this author's experience, effective DBS is a trade-off between effecting a sufficient neuronal response, most likely action potentials, in the intended targets versus spread of electrical stimulating current to unintended structures thereby causing side effects. Greater efficacy is generally associated with larger volumes and greater intensities (note that the two terms are not synonymous) so as to recruit more action potentials in more neural elements. However, avoidance of side effects may require electronically moving the stimulation electrical fields away from unintended structures by judicious choice of active electrode configurations or may necessitate smaller volumes and lesser intensities by combinations of electrical parameters and electrode configurations. There are electronic and electrophysiological properties that can be used to maneuver the stimulation electrical field as well as the distribution and intensities of the electrical fields.

Another principle to be exploited is that not all neural elements respond the same to the same DBS pulse as measured by the threshold to produce a neural response, specifically an action potential. Large diameter axons have lower thresholds than small diameter axons. Large diameter axons respond to narrower pulse widths than do small diameter axons. Axons have lower thresholds than dendrites, which have lower thresholds than cell bodies. Axonal terminals have the lowest threshold. Thus, variations in stimulation amplitudes and pulse widths can be exploited to narrow the response to only large diameter axons and axonal terminals or to expand the range of neural elements excited. Further, the orientation of the lines of electrical force that run from the negative electrode (cathode) to the positive electrode (anode) relative to the surface of the axonal membrane influences which axons are excited (Figure 4.1).

The basic unit of information in the brain

While neurons receive information in the form of synaptic inputs mediated by neurotransmitters and neuromodulators or in the form of electric gap junctions, the final product of neuronal processing is encoded in the sequence of action potentials that are conveyed down the axon to the next neuron (Figure 4.2). (There are a few types of neurons that do not use the all-or-nothing action potentials but rather a graded potential, such as the retinal bipolar cells.) Also, as described above, the main mechanism

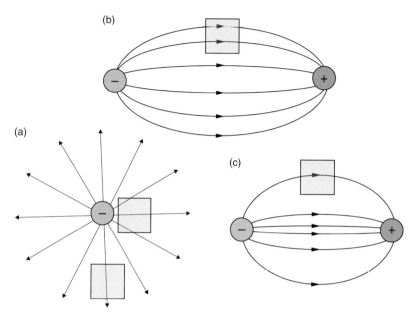

Figure 4.1 Schematic representation of the lines of electrical force that radiate from the negative electrode (cathode) for various configurations. In the case of monopolar (unipolar) configuration (a) where there is a single negative electrode (cathode) and a positive electrode (anode) a very far distance away (in electrical terms), as when the implanted neurostimulator metal case is used as the positive electrode, the lines of electrical force radiate out in all directions. In the case of bipolar configurations (b and c), where the negative electrode is near the positive electrode (on the same deep brain stimulation [DBS] lead), the lines of electrical force radiating out of the negative electrode are bent or pulled toward the positive electrode. The force or intensity of the electrical force can be conceptualized as the number of lines of electrical force that pass through a specific region of space, in this case represented by the box. As can be seen as the box moves away from the negative electrode (a), the lines of electrical force passing through the volume represented by the box get smaller, representing a reduction in the strength of the electrical field. In the case of the bipolar configuration, the geometry of the electrical field is more complicated. As can be seen in the wide bipolar configuration (b), there are a greater number of lines of electrical force further away from the line that connects the negative and positive contacts, as represented by the number of lines of electrical force passing through the volume represented by the shaded box compared to the narrow bipolar configuration. In the case of a narrow bipolar configuration (c), it is as though the closer positive electrode is pulling a greater number of lines of electrical force closer to the line that connects the negative and positive electrodes. This acts to pull them in from the space around the DBS lead, thereby reducing the intensity of the electrical fields at distances from the line connecting the negative and positive electrodes. Reproduced from Montgomery.[17]

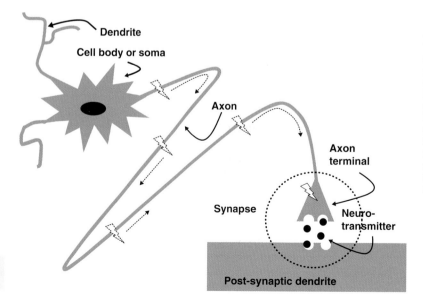

Figure 4.2 The neuron, consisting of a cell body, dendrites, axon, and axonal terminals leading to synaptic contacts on the next neuron. Once the neuronal membrane voltage reaches a depolarization threshold at the axon hillock (the beginning of the axon), an action potential is initiated (lightning bolt), which then proceeds down the axon to the synaptic terminal. There the action potential depolarizes the axon terminal, causing the release of neurotransmitters that initiate a change in the neuronal membrane potential in the dendrites or cell body of the next neuron.

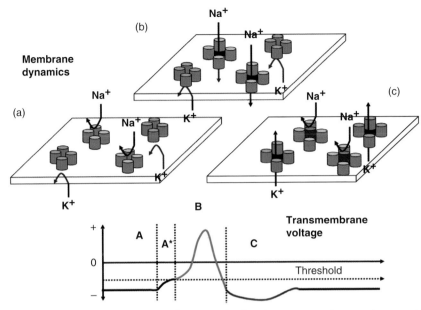

Membrane dynamics

Transmembrane voltage

Threshold

Figure 4.3 Schematic representation of one example of mechanisms generating an action potential. During the resting phase, the neuron pumps Na^+ ions out of the cell and K^+ ions into the cell. Relatively more Na^+ ions are pumped out compared to the number of K^+ ions that are pumped in. This results in the interior of the neuron having a negative voltage relative to the outside of the neuron (lower figure, segment A). Also, the difference in concentrations results in a driving force, pushing Na^+ inside and K^+ out. However, the flow of these ions is blocked at rest because the channels that allow the ions to move across the membrane are closed. (a) In response to excitation, the membrane voltage raises (lower figure, segment A*). Once a threshold is reached, the Na^+ channels open, allowing Na^+ ions to enter the neuron (b) and causing the neuronal membrane to become more positive (lower figure, segment B). Then the Na^+ channels become inactivated, thereby blocking further Na^+ ions from entering the neuron. Shortly afterwards, the K^+ ion channels open, allowing K^+ ions to flow out of the neuron (c), thus causing the membrane potential to become more negative and reversing the effects of the previous flow of Na^+ ions (lower figure, segment C). In fact, the efflux of K^+ ions temporarily makes the neuronal membrane relatively more negative than when the neuron is at rest resulting in a hyperpolarized state. The pumping mechanisms described above then restore the normal neuronal membrane potential at rest. Reproduced from Montgomery.[17]

of action of DBS probably relates to the action potentials generated in response to the DBS pulse. Consequently, it is worthwhile to understand the nature of the action potential.

An action potential could be considered analogous to an electrical spark or the light flash of a light bulb which are, in effect, flows of electrical current. In the case of an electrical spark or the flash of light, the flow of electricity is mediated by electrons, but in the case of a neuron, the electrical current is mediated by the flow of positively and negatively charged ions, such as sodium (Na^+), potassium (K^+), chloride (Cl^-), and calcium (Ca^{2+}).

In order for there to be a flow of electrical current, there must be some force to push the electrical current. Neurons create this force by creating an electrical potential across the cell membrane of the neuron. Neurons create a relatively greater positive charge outside the neuronal membrane and a relatively greater negative charge inside the neuron. The difference between the positivity outside the neuron

and the negativity inside the neuron is the membrane potential. Neurons create the membrane potential by pumping more positive ions, for example Na^+, out compared to the number of positive ions that are pumped in, for example K^+ (Figure 4.3). Note that this energy-dependent pumping also creates a concentration gradient, with relatively more Na^+ outside the neuron and more K^+ inside the neuron. This difference in concentration creates a force that, if allowed to act, would drive Na^+ ions into the neuron and K^+ ions out of the neuron. This force is the origin of the force that drives electrical current typified by the action potential.

For a spark to occur or for the light bulb to flash, a switch must be closed. Closing the switch allows electrons to flow through a gap to produce an electrical spark or to flow through the wire in the light bulb, which heats up to produce the flash of light. In the case of the neuron, the switch is in the neuronal membrane. In the electronic switch, a gap is closed between two conductors to let electrons flow through.

In the neuron, channels in the neuronal membrane open to allow ions to flow through (Figure 4.3).

In the case of an electrical spark or the light bulb, the electronic switch would need to be pushed closed to allow electrons to flow. In the neuron, the channels open to allow ions to flow or close to prevent ions from flowing, depending on the neuronal membrane potential. At rest the neuronal membrane potential may be -60 to -70 millivolts (mV). If the neuronal membrane potential decreases by becoming less negative (or more positive) it is depolarized. If the depolarization reaches a threshold the channels open allowing ions, such as Na^+ and K^+, to flow, generating an electrical flow or current. The time course of the Na^+ channels opening is much faster than the K^+ channels. The result is that Na^+ enters the neuron and the inside of the neuron becomes even less negative and finally becomes positive, transiently.

The influx of Na^+ is limited. When the neuronal membrane potential continues to decrease, becoming less negative, the Na^+ channels inactivate, preventing further flow of Na^+ ions and preventing the inside of the neuron from becoming more positive. The K^+ channels continue to be open and more positive ions leave, making the inside of the neuron more negative and thereby reversing the change in the neuronal membrane potential initiated by the flow of Na^+ ions into the neuron. When the neuronal membrane becomes more negative than the resting condition, the neuron is hyperpolarized. This hyperpolarization takes the neuronal membrane potential further away from the threshold, making it less likely to generate an action potential. This period of decreased excitability is called a relative refractory period. Also, the hyperpolarization deactivates the Na^+ channels, and until the Na^+ channels are reactivated, the neuron cannot generate an action potential. For the DBS pulse to initiate an action potential, the DBS pulse must depolarize the neuronal membrane, that is, reduce the difference between the relative positivity outside the neuron and the relative negativity inside the neuron. The DBS pulse can do so by dumping negative charges onto the outside of the neuron. The electrons exiting the DBS electrode during the DBS pulse are converted to negatively charged ions.

The key in DBS programming will be to control the spatial distribution and intensity of the electrical field generated by the DBS pulse that drives the negative ions onto the neuron.

A brief mention of depolarization blockade should be made because it has been offered as a potential mechanism of action of DBS. If the neuronal membrane is made less negative, or depolarized, but kept below the threshold for an action potential, Na^+ channels begin to close, thereby reducing the ability of the neuron to generate an action potential. However, there is considerable empirical evidence[3] as well as information from computational modeling[10] suggesting that depolarization blockade is not likely to be a mechanism of therapeutic action.

The electronics of DBS

The key to effective DBS is to control the number and spatial extent of neural elements in which action potentials are generated. Note that the number and spatial extent are not synonymous. For example, as will be demonstrated subsequently, a monopolar (unipolar) configuration – in which there is a single negative electrode (cathode) and the metal case of the implanted neurostimulator acts as the positive electrode (anode) – may generate a less intense but larger electrical field and activate fewer neural elements than a bipolar configuration, which though smaller in extent, is more intense.

The activation of neural elements will depend on the concentration of negative charges generated at the negative electrode (cathode), which will depend on how many electrons are being dumped by the cathode per unit time over the time of the DBS pulse. The measure of the number of electrons per unit time is *electrical current* and it is measured in amperes – typically in DBS, in milliamps. The total amount of electrons deposited is measured in coulombs, in DBS as microcoulombs. The force that drives the electrons out of the DBS negative electrode (cathode) is the *electromotive force* (EMF) and is measured in volts. The amount of electrical current delivered will depend on the amount of electromotive force, or voltage, and the resistance to the flow of electrical current. In the case of DBS, the resistance varies because the electrical current is not constant for each DBS pulse; rather, the current goes up and down rapidly. The resistance in such situations of fluctuating electrical current is called *impedance* and is measured in ohms.

Note that the impedance of the electrode is a function of the frequency components within the DBS pulse and not the frequency at which the pulses are delivered.

> The relationship between electrical current (I), electromotive force (E), and impedance (R) is given by Ohm's law: I = E/R.

This relationship is fundamentally important in DBS because the impedances, electromotive force (volts), and electrical current can vary between patients, between different stimulation parameters, with different configurations of active electrodes, and with the type of neurostimulator used. For example, the electrical current delivered by constant-voltage neurostimulators, which are designed to deliver a constant voltage regardless of the amount of electrical current, will be different because of differences in impedance – despite the same voltage. Constant-current neurostimulators automatically adjust the voltage as necessary for different impedances to maintain the same electrical current. The distinction is critical, as it is the electrical current delivered by the DBS pulse that determines the activation of neural elements. Also, it is the electrical current that figures in DBS safety and not the voltage.

Understanding these concepts often is facilitated by considering an analogy between the flow of electrons and the flow of water. Consider a water reservoir on a tower with a hose exiting from the bottom. The amount of water in the reservoir represents the stored electrical charges in the neurostimulator battery. One can think of electrical charge as the number of positive or negative ions or the number of electrons. The hose represents the DBS electrodes through which the electrons would flow. The water pressure in the hose depends on the height of the water reservoir, which would be analogous to the electromotive force or voltage. Higher towers are associated with higher water pressures and by analogy, voltages. The increased height of the water tower or higher voltage results in higher flows of water or electrical current, assuming the impedance (resistance) is constant. The amount of water delivered through the hose would correspond to the electrical charge measured in microcoulombs. The amount of water per unit time from the hose would correspond to the electrical current in milliamps. As common experience shows, smaller diameter hoses result in more resistance (impedance) to the flow of water. In this case the diameter of the hose would be inversely proportional to the impedance in the DBS system by analogy.

Manipulations of the water analogy help to understand the manipulations of the electronics in the DBS system. Picture the water tower at one height. There will be a certain hydrostatic force that will cause water to flow from the hose. Now picture the water tower rising to a new height. This will result in more force to move the water out of the hose. The increase in the height of the water tower would correspond to increasing the voltage. The result will be increased electrical current and deposition of more electrical charges during the stimulation pulse. Now consider the situation where the height of the water reservoir is constant but the diameter of the water hose increases, thereby reducing the impedance. The result will be a greater flow of water and more water delivered. By analogy, if the voltage remains constant but the impedance is reduced, there will be greater electrical current from the DBS electrode and greater amounts of electrical charges deposited in the brain. If the voltage is constant and the impedance increased, there will be less electrical current flowing into the brain.

> As previously stated, the electrical current, rather than voltage, has greater influence in causing an action potential in the neural elements. However, the actual factor is the electrical charge density, which is related to the rate by which electrical charges are injected into the brain (milliamps), the time period that the current flows (pulse width in DBS), and the surface area of the electrode. The relationship is give by the following equations.
>
> For constant-current neurostimulators:
>
> Charge density = (milliamps) * (pulse width)/ (surface area)
>
> For constant-voltage neurostimulators:
>
> Charge density = (volts/impedance) * (pulse width)/ (surface area)

Electrical current density at any one location distant from the electrode contact also depends on spread of the electrical charges through the tissue, the stimulation current (or the combination of voltage and electrode impedance), and the configuration of active electrodes (which DBS contacts are anodes and cathodes). The tissue affords impedance to the flow of electrical charges, just like the water hose. The tissue impedance depends on the makeup of the tissue; for example, gray matter affords less imped-ance than does white matter. Thus, the regional anat-omy surrounding the DBS electrodes influences how far and in what direction the electrical charges will flow. Usually, the effects of the tissue impedances are not controllable by the user. However, the other factors (such as stimulation current or the voltage in the voltage/impedance combination) and the elec-trode configurations are controllable.

Constant-voltage versus constant-current neurostimulators

The control of the stimulating current is quite differ-ent in constant-current versus constant-voltage devices. The stimulating current is directly controlled by the constant-current neurostimulator. As the impedance changes, the device automatically adjusts the voltage, as per Ohm's Law, to maintain the same stimulation current. With constant-voltage neurosti-mulators, the changing impedances will result in dif-ferent stimulation currents. Thus, if the impedances change (even if the voltage is constant), there will be a change in the stimulation currents and, consequently, a different physiological and possibly clinical effect.

The relative advantage of a constant-current neuro-stimulator versus a constant-voltage device depends on how much the electrode impedances change. In DBS patients, it seems that initially following implant-ation, there may indeed be changes in the impedance. However, over months, there may not be significant changes. Thus, the clinical benefit of a constant-current device is unclear. While the impedances may be constant within a single subject, though, the impedances may differ greatly between subjects.[11] This means that DBS at a certain voltage in one patient may have different clinical effects compared to the same voltage in another patient. This makes it difficult to generalize across patients or draw comparisons between patients.

Active electrode configurations

The electrical charge generated during the DBS pulse dissipates with distance from the electrode. The elec-trical charge is highest near the active electrode con-tact. The spatial extent of the spread of the electrical charge is directly proportional to the stimulation cur-rent (or voltage/impedance combination). Thus, the electrical charge per unit volume of tissue gets less as the distance from the electrode increases. The elec-trical charge per unit volume is known as the elec-trical charge density, which is the critical factor determining the neuronal response to DBS and safety. The charge density also is greatly affected by the configuration of active electrodes.

Configurations of active electrodes can be grouped into monopolar (also called unipolar) and bipolar or multi-polar. In the multi-polar configur-ations there are one or more cathodes (negative elec-trodes) and one or more anodes (positive electrodes). A bipolar configuration is a multi-polar configuration where a single electrode is negatively charged and the other is positively charged. In monopolar configur-ations, there are one or more negative electrodes on the DBS lead, while the positive electrode is on the neurostimulator case. In monopolar configurations, the distance between the negative and positive elec-trodes is considered infinite. In the case of multi-polar configurations, the negative and positive electrodes are relatively close to each other. Whereas in the bipolar configuration, the electrical current flow is directed from the cathode to the anode, in the mono-polar configuration, the electrical charge flows out in all directions from the cathode because the anode is considered to be "infinitely" distant.

For monopolar DBS, the intensity of the electrical field falls off in proportion to the distance from the electrode. A doubling of the distance will reduce the intensity to half. However, for bipolar configurations, doubling the distance will reduce the intensity to one-quarter. A tripolar configuration, consisting of a negative electrode bracketed by two adjacent positive electrodes (one on each side), will reduce the intensity to one-eighth when the distance is doubled. Thus, if one were to plot iso-intensity fields (contours that mark the same intensities), the electrical field would be larger with the monopolar, smaller with the bipo-lar, and smallest with the tripolar.

The distance between the positive electrode and the negative electrode also affects the intensity of the elec-tric field (Figure 4.1). The intensity increases as the square of the distance between the electrodes. Thus, doubling the distance between the negative and posi-tive electrodes increases the intensity by a factor of four. Wide bipolar configurations will give a higher intensity electric field compared to a narrow bipolar. For those reasons, use of DBS leads with wider spaced electrodes (such as the Medtronic model 3387 DBS lead) will allow generation of more intense fields compared to DBS leads with more narrowly spaced electrodes (such as the Medtronic model 3389). Which and how many axons can be stimulated to produce an action potential can be controlled by the stimulation current (or voltage/impedance). Increasing the current or voltage (the latter assuming a constant impedance) can stimulate action potentials in more axons based on increasing the spatial extent of the electrical field intensities. Within the electrical field, increasing stimulation currents or voltages (the latter assuming constant impedance) also increases the number of axons stimulated, since axons of different sizes have different thresholds. Initially, large diameter axons are recruited at lower currents or voltages and progressively smaller axons are recruited as the currents and voltages are increased.

The width of the DBS pulse also can be used to control which axons are excited to produce action potentials. Large diameter axons can be excited by short pulse widths, and small diameter axons require longer pulse widths.

Putting it together

The stimulation parameters and electrode configurations can be used to control the spatial extent and number of axons excited by the DBS pulse. These factors can be exploited to increase efficacy, perhaps by increasing the number of axons excited within the DBS target. Further, these factors can be exploited to prevent excitation of axons that would result in side effects.

Consider the example shown in Figure 4.4. In this case, the subthalamic nucleus (STN) or globus pallidus internus (GPi) is the intended target, but the corticospinal tract lies in the adjacent internal capsule. The goal is to activate sufficient axons from, to, or passing through the STN or GPi without exciting action potentials in the axons of the corticospinal tract in the internal capsule. In Figure 4.4a, monopolar DBS is used and only the two larger axons are excited in GPi or STN. In order to increase the number of axons excited, the stimulation current or voltage can be increased, as in Figure 4.4b. While this increases the number of axons excited in GPi or STN, the increased current or voltage activates axons in the internal capsule, leading to tonic muscle contraction as a side effect. An alternative would be to change the configuration to move the higher current or voltage negative electrode way from the internal capsule (Figure 4.4d), but this may not be feasible. Another option would be to

stimulate using a bipolar configuration, which shrinks the electrical field and directs the field away from the internal capsule, as shown in Figure 4.4c. Finally, one could use the original monopolar configuration and current or voltage associated with Figure 4.4a but use a longer pulse width that increases the number of axons activated by recruiting smaller diameter axons (Figure 4.4e).

DBS rate

The effects of varying the rate (frequency) of DBS on neuronal activities are less straightforward. Previously it was thought that high frequency DBS inhibits the stimulated target and low frequency excites the target.[12] In the past, high frequency DBS was thought therapeutic, while low frequency stimulation exacerbated symptoms and signs. However, it is now clear that low frequency DBS may be therapeutic as well. Further, neurophysiological studies involving microelectrode recordings in various nuclei of the basal ganglia–thalamic–cortical system in response to STN DBS in non-human primates demonstrate no qualitative differences in neuronal responses to different frequencies of STN DBS. Rather, there are quantitative differences.[3] For example, only the magnitude of response changes and is greater with high frequency stimulation, for example at 130 Hz.

One possible explanation has been offered by the Systems Oscillators theory, which posits that the basal ganglia–thalamic–cortical system is organized as sets of nested, interconnected, reentrant, non-linear oscillators of different lengths and consequently different fundamental frequencies.[13–15] For example, the closed feedback loop comprised of the ventrolateral thalamus and motor cortex results in action potentials that traverse the closed circuit, hence reentrant oscillators. This disynaptic pathway is short and thus associated with a high inherent frequency approximating 147 Hz. The unique properties of the neurons, such as refractory periods and postinhibitory rebound excitability, confer non-linear properties that may be important to prevent run-away activity within the positive feedback loop comprised of the thalamo-cortical circuit.

Similarly, the basal ganglia–thalamic–cortical system also contains a closed feedback loop comprised of projections from motor cortex to putamen to globus pallidus externa (GPe) to GPi to thalamus to motor cortex. This circuit is much longer, and

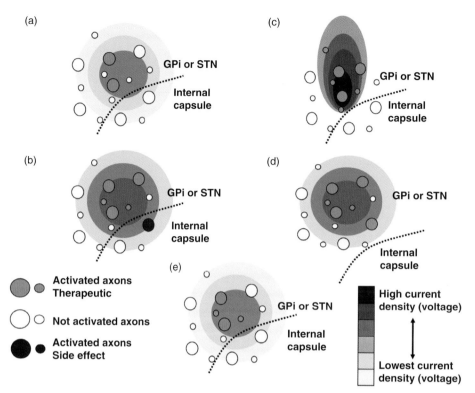

(a)

(c)

(b)

(d)

(e)

Activated axons
Therapeutic

Not activated axons

Activated axons
Side effect

High current
density (voltage)

Lowest current
density (voltage)

Figure 4.4 An hypothetical example of the effects of varying stimulation parameters and electrode configurations on the shape, size, and intensity of the electrical fields generated by the deep brain stimulation pulse. See text for explanation. Reproduced from Montgomery.[17]

reentrant activity would take longer to traverse this circuit and would result in a much lower frequency oscillation. These two circuits are linked through the thalamus and motor cortex, and the oscillatory activities within each circuit interact with each other.

The Systems Oscillators theory posits that DBS at specific frequencies results in resonance amplification of the inherent or fundamental frequency of the circuit or loop that is stimulated. Different symptoms and signs may depend on different circuits or loops and consequently be affected by different DBS frequencies.

How these theories of the effects of different DBS frequencies translate to DBS programming is problematic. Suffice it to say, one may have to pick some frequency in the lower range of those found to be effective for a specific symptom or sign in a specific disease and then assess different frequencies around that initial DBS frequency for clinical effect.

The "U-shaped" response

The "U-shaped" response is the observation that symptoms and signs can improve with increasing stimulation parameters until a certain point. Increasing these parameters beyond this point may worsen symptoms and signs.

> The practical implication for DBS programming is the importance of starting at lower values of stimulation parameters and increasing by small enough steps so as to not miss the optimal response.

The neurophysiological principles underlying the "U-shaped" response are unclear. One current hypothesis is that the resonance amplification of the underlying signal in the neuronal spike trains operates within a narrow band. Disease may reduce the probability of a neuronal discharge at the appropriate time, resulting in a loss of signal necessary to drive appropriate behaviors and thereby causing the symptoms and signs of disease.[16] One could imagine someone typing at a computer keyboard, with the sequence of different key strikes conveying the important information. Imagine that at random times, the typist fails to strike the appropriate key. There would be a loss of information and dysfunction. Therapeutic DBS may increase the probability of a key strike generically. Thus, increasing the probability leads to a greater probability that an intended key strike will take place, thus restoring information and more normal function. However, further increases in the generic or non-specific probability of a key strike now start to result in unintended key strikes, resulting in increasing misinformation and dysfunction.

Safety

Excessive stimulation can lead to tissue damage by several mechanisms. First, passing any electrical current through an impedance (resistance) will cause heat. Excessive current through the DBS lead could cause heating and tissue damage. The presently accepted safety limit is 30 microcoulombs/cm^2 per phase. Residual unbalanced charge left on the electrodes can cause hydrolysis with the formation of gas bubbles that can tear tissue. In addition, unbalanced charges can create other reactive chemical species that can cause tissue damage. The DBS clinician programmer monitors the stimulation parameters that are being proposed and alerts the clinician in advance if they are attempting to program stimulation parameters that could exceed the charge density safety limit and potentially cause tissue injury.

Implications for clinical care

Deep brain stimulation is remarkably effective, succeeding when all manner of other therapies have failed. As evidenced by the discussions in this chapter, the success of DBS therapy should not be a surprise. After all, the brain processes and conveys information electronically. The neurotransmitters, which are the basis for most pharmacological therapies, are the messengers – not the message. The experience with DBS demonstrates the importance and value of reconsidering neurological and psychiatric disorders as disorders of information, not of neurotransmitters.

On a more practical level, there is little question that currently accepted DBS therapies are underutilized. To be sure this may be due to overestimation of risk and underestimation of benefit. However, this author believes that another reason is the perceived "foreignness" of DBS. Clinicians often feel comfortable prescribing dangerous medications but are uncomfortable prescribing electricity. The intent of this chapter is to demonstrate that the electrophysiology underlying DBS is not mysterious. Effective postoperative DBS programming can be facilitated by knowledge of the underlying physiological principles, combined with knowledge of the regional anatomy.

References

1. Anderson ME, Postupna N, Ruffo M. Effects of high-frequency stimulation in the internal globus pallidus on the activity of thalamic neurons in the awake monkey. *J Neurophysiol* 2003;**89**:1150–60.

2. Hashimoto T, Elder CM, Okun MS, Patrick SK, Vitek JL. Stimulation of the subthalamic nucleus changes the firing pattern of pallidal neurons. *J Neurosci* 2003;**23**:1916–23.

3. Montgomery EB, Jr., Gare JT. Mechanisms of action of deep brain stimulation (DBS). *Neurosci Biobehav Rev* 2008;**32**:388–407.

4. Montgomery EB, Jr. Effects of GPi stimulation on human thalamic neuronal activity. *Clin Neurophysiol* 2006;**117**:2691–702.

5. Alterman RL, Miravite J, Weisz D, et al. Sixty Hertz pallidal deep brain stimulation for primary torsion dystonia. *Neurology* 2007;**69**:681–8.

6. Wojtecki L, Timmermann L, Jorgens S, et al. Frequency-dependent reciprocal modulation of verbal fluency and motor functions in subthalamic deep brain stimulation. *Arch Neurol* 2006;**63**:1273–6.

7. Lozano AM, Eltahawy H. How does DBS work? *Clin Neurophysiol* 2004;**57**:733–6.

8. Bekar L, Libionka W, Tian G, et al. Adenosine is crucial for deep brain stimulation-mediated attenuation of tremor. *Nat Med* 2008;**14**:75–80.

9. Olanow CW, Goetz CG, Kordower JH, et al. A double-blind controlled trial of bilateral fetal nigral transplantation in Parkinson's disease. *Ann Neurol* 2003;**54**:403–14.

10. McIntyre CC, Savasta M, Walter BL, Vitek JL. How does deep brain stimulation work? Present understanding and future questions. *J Clin Neurophysiol* 2004;**21**:40–50.

11. Sillay K, Montgomery EB, Jr. Therapeutic DBS electrode impedances: analysis with long-term follow-up. Annual meeting of the American Society for Stereotactic and Functional Neurosurgery; 2008.

12. Montgomery EB, Jr., Baker KB. Mechanisms of deep brain stimulation and future technical developments. *Neurol Res* 2000;**22**:259–66.

13. Montgomery EB, Jr. Dynamically coupled, high-frequency reentrant, non-linear oscillators

embedded in scale-free basal ganglia-thalamic-cortical networks mediating function and deep brain stimulation effects. *Nonlinear Studies* 2004;**11**:385–421.

14. Montgomery EB, Jr. Basal ganglia physiology and pathophysiology: a reappraisal. *Parkinsonism Relat Disord* 2007;**13**:455–65.

15. Montgomery EB, Jr. Theorizing about the role of the basal ganglia in speech and language: the epidemic of miss-reasoning and an alternative. *Comm Dis Rev* 2008;**2**:1–15.

16. Montgomery EB, Jr., Sillay K Nested probabilistic oscillators in DBS and basal ganglia function. Movement Disorders Society 12th Annual Meeting. Chicago; 2008.

17. Montgomery EB, Jr. *Deep Brain Stimulation Programming: Principles and Practice.* New York: Oxford University Press, 2010.

Chapter 5

Fundamentals of deep brain stimulation programming

S. Elizabeth Zauber, Peggie A. Smith, and Leo Verhagen Metman

Introduction

This chapter will serve as a brief guide for clinicians taking care of patients with implanted deep brain stimulation (DBS) systems. We will discuss general principles that apply to all patients, regardless of their disease or site of stimulation in their brain. Other chapters will focus on programming issues specific to essential tremor (ET) (Chapter 6), Parkinson's disease (PD) (Chapter 7), and dystonia (Chapter 8), while the basic electrical principles underlying DBS are discussed in depth in Chapter 4.

It is not unusual for healthcare providers to be hesitant to embrace the management of DBS patients, as a common impression is that programming the stimulation system is complicated, time consuming, and highly technical.

> Though it is undeniable that programming DBS systems requires patience and persistence, it is also true that by applying a systematic approach one can move away from an inefficient and time consuming process with unpredictable results toward an efficient, effective, and successful programming session.

In the following paragraphs we will first briefly describe the different components of available DBS systems that are relevant to the programmer. Next we will discuss the stimulation parameters that can be manipulated. Subsequently we will describe what will take place at the first postoperative visit when stimulation is initiated, and then what needs to be done during the follow-up programming visits. Before we proceed, it is important to emphasize that there are several different and valid programming strategies. Though the approach outlined below has been

successful in our environment and is commonly used by clinicians throughout the world, accumulated experience will lead programmers to develop variations that work best within their particular practice.

Hardware components

In order to understand the fundamentals of programming, it is important to be familiar with the devices used for DBS. In addition, basic knowledge of the different components of the DBS system will be important for troubleshooting, as discussed in Chapter 9. The implantable components of the system include the neurostimulator (also called an implantable neurostimulator [INS] or implantable pulse generator [IPG]), the quadripolar DBS lead, and an extension that connects the DBS lead to the neurostimulator (Figure 5.1). External instruments that interact with the device include the clinician programmer and the patient programmer (Figure 5.2).

Neurostimulator

The neurostimulator is a titanium unit containing the electronics and power supply of the DBS system (Figure 5.3). It is implanted in a subcutaneous pocket, usually located under the clavicle but alternatively in the abdomen. Three major types of neurostimulators are currently available in the United States and worldwide: a single channel, primary cell (non-rechargeable) model (Soletra, Medtronic, Inc.); dual channel primary cell models (Kinetra and Activa PC, Medtronic, Inc.); and a dual channel rechargeable model (Activa RC, Medtronic, Inc.). In Europe, two additional neurostimulators are available: a single channel, primary cell (non-rechargeable) model (Libra, St. Jude Medical, Inc.) and a dual channel primary cell model (Libra XP, St. Jude Medical, Inc.).

Deep Brain Stimulation Management, ed. William J. Marks, Jr. Published by Cambridge University Press.
© Cambridge University Press 2011.

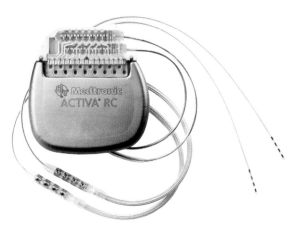

Figure 5.1 Deep brain stimulation (DBS) system, including a neurostimulator, extensions, and DBS leads. Figure courtesy of Medtronic, Inc.; used with permission.

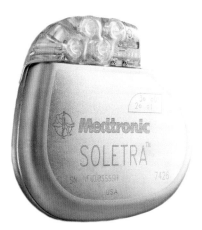

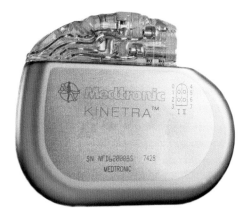

Figure 5.3 Deep brain stimulation neurostimulators. Figures courtesy of Medtronic, Inc., and St. Jude Medical, Inc.; used with permission.

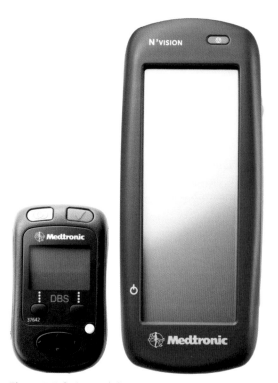

Figure 5.2 Patient and clinician programmers. Figure courtesy of Medtronic, Inc.; used with permission.

Single channel neurostimulators

These devices provide stimulation to one DBS lead, treating a target in one hemisphere of the brain. Patients requiring bilateral DBS treatment, and therefore two DBS leads, will thus need two single channel neurostimulators. Usually one is placed under each clavicle. Intuitively, it may seem advantageous to have only one (dual channel) neurostimulator, but there are some potential advantages to using two separate devices in a patient. The smaller size of the single channel device may be more comfortable for small or thin patients than a dual channel primary cell device. Further, if the device

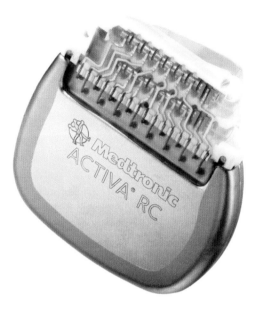
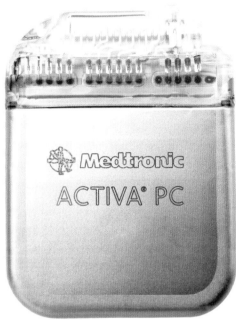
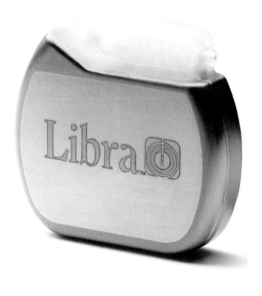
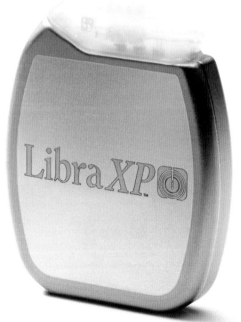

Figure 5.3 *(cont.)*

fails or needs to be removed due to infection, patients who originally had two neurostimulators can receive at least some benefit from the remaining contralateral neurostimulator.

Dual channel neurostimulators

Dual channel neurostimulators deliver stimulation to two separate DBS leads, enabling bilateral therapy. Implanting only one neurostimulator, rather than two, may be surgically advantageous, since fewer incisions and less tunneling of extensions is required. In order to provide sufficient power, however, a larger primary (non-rechargeable) battery within the neurostimulator is required, thus resulting in a larger size device. The rechargeable dual channel neurostimulator addresses this issue by providing bilateral stimulation in a compact device. In order to achieve the small device size and prolonged battery longevity afforded by a rechargeable system, patients using such a device are required to recharge their neurostimulator battery on a regular (generally weekly) basis for the life of the device. This requirement may not be well suited for patients with cognitive or motor impairment or those without access to caregiver assistance. Because primary cell devices do not require maintenance by the patient, they are better suited to patients with these issues or in those who simply want a maintenance-free experience. Dual channel devices, whether rechargeable or not, also require that the same rate of stimulation be used for each hemisphere; this is generally not a clinically meaningful limitation, but occasionally patients may benefit from the ability to assign different stimulation rates on each side to optimize symptom control.

Quadripolar DBS leads

Presently in the United States two different DBS leads are available (Figure 5.4). Both leads contain four platinum/iridium electrodes encased in a polymer-based insulation. Both leads measure 1.27 mm in diameter and have individual electrodes that are 1.5 mm in length. The difference between the two lead models is due to the spacing between each of the four electrodes, with one model (Medtronic model 3387) having inter-electrode spacing of 1.5 mm (providing a total span of 10.5 mm with which to stimulate) and the other (Medtronic model 3389) having 0.5 mm inter-electrode spacing

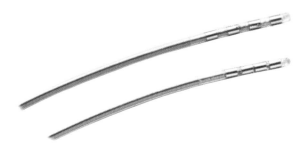

Figure 5.4 Deep brain stimulation leads. Figure courtesy of Medtronic, Inc.; used with permission.

(providing a total span of 7.5 mm). Either lead can be used for stimulation in the usual targets to treat movement disorders, but often the lead with the wider span is used for larger targets (ventral intermediate nucleus of the thalamus [Vim] or globus pallidus internus [GPi]) and the lead with the smaller span for the smaller target ([STN]).

Extensions

The extension, a small-diameter wire cable encased in silicone insulation, is used to connect each DBS lead to the neurostimulator (Figure 5.1). The extension, which is tunneled under the skin, attaches to the DBS lead via a connector that is usually placed above the mastoid region. Extensions are available in different lengths to accommodate different body sizes and placement of the neurostimulator in either the chest or abdominal area.

Clinician programmer

This portable device (for example, Medtronic model 8840, Figure 5.2) is used by clinicians to communicate wirelessly with the neurostimulator using radio-frequency telemetry. Using a programming wand, the clinician uses the programmer to stipulate electrode configurations, to adjust the various stimulation parameters, and to activate various features of the DBS system.

Patient programmers

These instruments serve as portable "remote controls" to be used by patients and their caregivers to interact with their neurostimulators (Figure 5.2). Depending on the model of the neurostimulator and its associated patient programmer, patients may be able to turn on and off their device, check the battery status of their device, adjust stimulation parameter levels within clinician-specified ranges, select from among different groups of stimulation settings, and (for a rechargeable neurostimulator) ascertain the battery charge status.

Adjustability of DBS

In order to optimize the effects of DBS by providing maximal symptom suppression without unacceptable stimulation-induced adverse effects, clinicians can modify the electrode configuration and the electrical parameters used to deliver stimulation. Elements of electrode configuration include designating which electrode(s) on the DBS system are active and the arrangement of electrode polarity (assigning the negative and positive electrodes) (Figure 5.5). Stimulation

parameters that can be adjusted include the amplitude, pulse width, and rate (Figure 5.6).

Electrode configuration

There are four electrodes per lead that can be used as the active electrode, alone or in combination. The clinician determines which electrode(s) provides the best relief of symptoms (as described below) to the patient, with the active electrode producing clinical benefit assigned to have a negative polarity (that is, to serve as the cathode).

In addition to selecting the negative electrode(s), the clinician also has a choice designating the positive electrode(s) (the anode) (Figure 5.6). With monopolar (also known as unipolar) stimulation, the metal case of the neurostimulator is designated

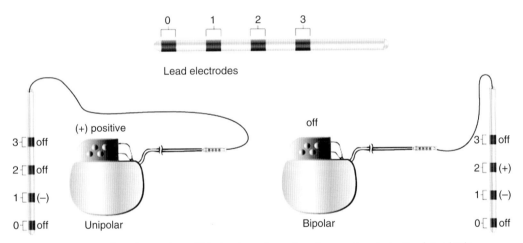

Figure 5.5 Example of simple unipolar and bipolar electrode configurations on deep brain stimulation leads.

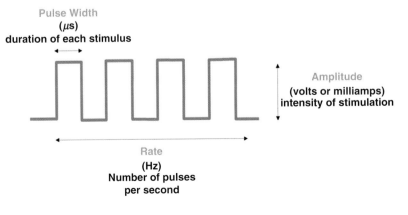

Figure 5.6 Stimulation parameters for deep brain stimulation.

as the positive electrode. With bipolar stimulation, the case is not active; instead, one (or more) of the remaining electrodes on the DBS lead serves as the positive electrode. Monopolar stimulation creates a spherical area of stimulation around the negative electrode, whereas bipolar stimulation creates a more elongated but constricted field between the two selected electrodes. The clinician can take advantage of the more focused stimulation of the bipolar configuration to limit spread of the field and therefore reduce side effects of stimulating structures adjacent to the intended stimulation target.

Amplitude

> The amplitude is the main parameter used to control the intensity of stimulation.

Increasing the amplitude will cause further spread of the field of stimulation, affecting neural elements at increasing distances from the electrode. It is estimated that at usual settings the electrical current diffuses about 3 mm radially from the electrode. Historically, DBS devices have operated as constant-voltage devices, in which the amplitude of stimulation is controlled by adjusting voltage. The voltage can be adjusted in small increments (usually in 0.1 volt (V) steps), between 0 and 10.5 V. Newer devices (Activa RC and Activa PC, Medtronic, Inc.) can also be used in a constant-current mode, in which the amplitude is regulated by adjusting the current, with the ability to set the amplitude between 0 and 25.5 milliamps (mA). Additional devices operate only in the constant current mode (Libra and Libra XP, St. Jude Medical, Inc.).

Pulse width

> Pulse width refers to the duration of each electrical pulse delivered.

Increasing the pulse width will excite more and different neuronal elements within the same volume of tissue. Usually a pulse width of 60 or 90 microseconds (μs) is chosen initially, and increased if needed (with the maximum pulse width being 450 μs).

Rate

In general, the efficacy of DBS is based on high frequency stimulation. Frequencies (or rates) below 50 pulses per second (pps) or Hertz (Hz) are typically not efficacious for most conditions with stimulation of typical brain targets and can actually cause stimulation-induced worsening of tremor and other symptoms.

> In most patients with PD and ET, the rate of stimulation is usually ≥ 130 Hz. In many instances, further rate increases will not offer substantial additional benefit.

A minority of patients, however, will respond to higher rates of stimulation, especially in the case of recalcitrant tremor. The maximal rate that can be programmed varies with the device and is either 185 Hz or 250 Hz. Most commonly used rates are between 130 and 185 Hz for PD and ET, whereas the situation may be more variable for dystonia, with some patients responding to lower rates (50–60 Hz) of stimulation (see Chapter 8).

Initial visit (Table 5.1)
Preparation
Timing

Most centers wait 3–4 weeks after implantation of the DBS leads to initiate stimulation. Insertion of the leads often causes a transient improvement in symptoms, called a "micro-lesion" effect. Waiting to perform initial DBS programming until this transient improvement subsides and symptoms of parkinsonism, tremor, or dystonia have returned makes it easier to assess benefit from stimulation.

Duration

Clinicians should set aside at least 30–60 minutes per DBS lead for initial programming. This time period provides a good compromise between longer sessions, which lead to patient fatigue, and shorter sessions, which may not allow for adequate observation during electrode screening and for patient education.

Medication state

Patients with PD should arrive for initial (and sometimes subsequent) programming sessions

Table 5.1 Initial programming checklist

Before visit

- Review postoperative imaging
- Review intraoperative records
- Contact patient with instructions

At visit

Before programming

Take interval history

- Surgical side effects

  cognition, mood

  microlesion effect

- Motor symptoms
- Dyskinesia exacerbation (for PD patients)
- Medication changes

Perform physical exam

- Skin incisions

Neurological exam

- Choose a motor sign to follow

Explain the programming process

Programming

- Perform electrode impedance check
- Set pulse width (60–90 µs) and rate (130–185 Hz)
- Perform monopolar review of each electrode
- Assess therapeutic window
- Select optimal electrode(s) and refine stimulation parameters
- Reset counters
- Document final settings

After programming

- Educate patient on use of patient programmer
- Educate patient on safety issues
- Decide on any medication changes that may need to be implemented

Note: PD, Parkinson's disease.

without medications (particularly levodopa) in effect, as the presence of medication often obscures the ability to evaluate the effects of the stimulation itself on parkinsonian signs and symptoms. Some clinicians suggest that patients withhold anti-parkinsonian medication for 12 hours, to produce a "practically defined off state," but it is usually sufficient to hold 1–2 doses of medication preceding the programming session. Programming in the "off" state allows the symptoms of PD to be evident so that the effect of stimulation can be observed. Patients with ET or dystonia should take their usual medications, since their movement disorder symptoms would be expected to be evident even on medication.

Participants

We recommend that patients bring a friend or family member to the first programming session. This provides support to the patient, helps in assessing changes in the patient's function, and assists in the educational process. More than one or two family members or the presence of small children may be a distraction, however, and should be discouraged. Patients should also bring their patient programmer and their current medication schedule, since medication adjustments are often discussed.

Surgical and imaging data

The programming clinician should communicate with the surgeon to know which DBS lead has been implanted. It may also be helpful to review the results of intraoperative stimulation and postoperative MRI findings, since this information can help programmers understand and anticipate the beneficial effects and side effects of stimulation.

Documentation

Record keeping is an essential aspect of DBS programming, and most clinicians use dedicated forms to organize their programming data. This ensures that the programming process proceeds in an organized manner and prevents inadvertent duplication of previously unsuccessful device settings. Documentation for each programming session should include entry and exit parameters, the reason for changes, and the clinical response (beneficial and adverse effects) to settings. Device diagnostic information, such as impedance measurements and battery voltage, should be documented as well. Several templates have been developed as guidelines, but clinicians should modify them into a format that works best for them (Appendices I–K). In addition to a record of each programming session, it is helpful to have a second form that summarizes the final electrode configuration and stimulation parameters at the end of each visit and the reason for any changes that were made. Such a document enables the clinician to quickly review prior settings (Appendix L).

Interval history

The clinician should review how the patient has been recovering from surgery, whether there has been a change in behavior or cognition, and whether there has been a "micro-lesion" effect causing improvement in symptoms.

Physical exam

The clinician will perform a brief neurological exam, including inspection of the surgical incisions to ensure adequate wound healing and identify, if present, any signs of developing infection.

Selecting a sign or symptom to assess

> During programming sessions, it will not be practical to repeatedly perform a full motor examination (nor is that necessary). Instead, programming clinicians should choose one or two clinical signs to follow for each individual patient.

Essential tremor patients often display the most tremor when drawing a spiral or pouring water, and these activities can be used to evaluate tremor severity during programming. In patients with PD, though, tremor is not always the most reliable sign because it may be intermittent and influenced by anxiety. In a patient with severe, persistent tremor, this sign can be very useful to gauge when effective DBS settings have been attained. Bradykinesia can also serve as a sign to assess and follow, especially when a quantitative measure is available (such as the number of movement repetitions per unit of time), but the task should be simple and quick to avoid fatigue.

> Rigidity of the wrist or elbow is usually an extremely helpful sign to assess in patients with PD, because it improves quickly with stimulation and is not dependent on patient effort.

Of course clinicians programming DBS should not just evaluate one sign; they should also consider the entire clinical picture. From time to time patients should be asked to stand and walk, allowing observation of improved arm swing that can be a sensitive sign of decreased bradykinesia and because subtle stimulation-related side effects, such as spread of stimulation to internal capsule, may be detected when observing gait. In dystonia, most of the initial programming is focused on assessing for stimulation-related adverse effects, rather than on benefit, because improvement usually does not occur acutely but instead develops over days to months (see Chapter 8).

Choosing sides

It is preferable to begin programming the DBS lead contralateral to the side with the most severe symptoms first, since benefit may be more obvious and also welcome to the patient. Once DBS on one side is programmed, stimulation can be kept on and attention then turned to the opposite side. Alternatively, the programming clinician may choose to program each side individually, with stimulation on the opposite side turned off. In this case, it should be recognized that with bilateral stimulation there may be additive effects, both beneficial and adverse, that ultimately will need to be assessed.

Explanation of the process

> The main goal of the initial programming visit is to determine the best therapeutic electrode(s) for chronic stimulation. This is accomplished by carefully screening each electrode with test stimulation to determine the amplitude thresholds for beneficial and adverse effects at each electrode.

It is important to communicate this goal to patients so that they understand that side effects are expected and, in fact, are intentionally induced. They should be reassured that side effects will be mild and rapidly reversible.

Programming
Check impedances

Before proceeding with programming the DBS system, a complete diagnostic impedance check should be performed and documented at the initial visit to confirm the integrity of the hardware and establish a baseline for the individual patient. The clinician programmer automates this process, providing monopolar and bipolar impedance values for each electrode and combination of electrodes. Each device has specific ranges of normal operating impedances. Abnormally high impedances suggest a discontinuity along the DBS system ("open circuit"). In the initial postoperative period, high impedances may result from damage to the DBS lead or extension during the procedure, or a suboptimal connection of the extension to either the neurostimulator or to the DBS lead. Later on, newly detected high impedances associated with loss of efficacy should raise the suspicion for wire fracture of the lead or extension, especially when preceded by trauma. A fracture can be confirmed with X-rays of the skull, neck, and chest (often referred to as a "shunt series" since used to assess ventriculoperitoneal shunts). Conversely, low impedances can indicate a short circuit. Clinicians encountering these issues can enlist the assistance of technical support services provided by the device manufacturer.

Screen the electrodes for effects

It is important to minimize variables during the process of electrode selection to allow clear identification of electrodes that are well located and provide the best therapeutic benefit. Therefore pulse width and rate should be set and not changed so that amplitude is the only parameter being changed and explored at each electrode. A pulse width of 60 μs and a frequency of 130 Hz are appropriate initial settings; see individual chapters for more details of these settings for all indications.

> Monopolar screening (or review) of electrodes is a term that refers to the clinician's systematic exploration of stimulation-induced benefits and side effects at each electrode.

Starting with the most ventral (lowest) contact, which is configured to be negative while the neurostimulator case is set as the positive electrode, stimulation amplitude is increased gradually. The amplitude at which clinical improvement occurs is noted, as well as the amplitude at which persistent stimulation-induced adverse effects occur.

> Amplitude should, in fact, be increased until a stimulation-related side effect occurs, even if this requires an amplitude higher than would be used clinically, because the threshold for the occurrence of side effects will provide information about the therapeutic window at each electrode and give an impression of the electrode location relative to surrounding neural structures.

Once amplitude-limiting side effects have occurred at a given electrode, the next electrode on the DBS lead should be explored in a similar fashion. This process should be continued until all four electrodes have been assessed. The nature of possible side effects varies depending on the DBS target (STN, Vim, GPi), further described in the relevant later chapters.

> The electrode with the largest therapeutic window (difference between thresholds for efficacy and adverse effects) is the one typically selected for chronic stimulation (Figure 5.7).

If two adjacent electrodes appear equally suited for chronic stimulation, one approach is to choose one electrode for the first month of stimulation (for example, electrode 1 in the monopolar mode) and then select the other (for example, electrode 2 in the

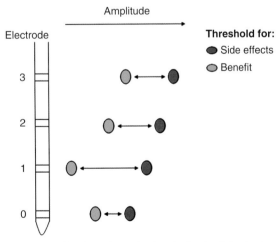

Figure 5.7 The electrode on the deep brain stimulation lead providing the largest therapeutic window is usually the best to use for chronic stimulation. In this example, electrode 1 has the largest therapeutic window, defined by the greatest span between the amplitude thresholds for stimulation-related benefits and stimulation-induced adverse effects.

monopolar mode) at the next visit to allow the patient to determine which of the two electrodes provides the best motor function in the home environment. If this strategy is followed, other stimulation parameters and medications should not be changed during this evaluation period whenever possible in order to avoid confounding assessment of the best therapeutic electrode. Another approach is to stimulate through both electrodes (for example, using both electrodes 1 and 2 as negative electrodes in the monopolar mode), since this may provide additive benefit. In this case, since the stimulation field will be increased, it may be possible (or necessary) to lower the stimulation intensity. If no single electrode can provide therapeutic benefit *without* side effects in the monopolar mode, then the more focused bipolar mode may provide a valuable alternative.

> For bipolar stimulation, the electrode to be assigned negative polarity will be the one that was most effective during monopolar review, while the electrode to be designated as positive can be any of the three remaining contacts.

A good initial choice for the positive electrode is the one that was associated with some beneficial effects during monopolar review. The shape of the electrical field depends on which electrode configuration is chosen.

Set the amplitude

Once the best electrode(s) is chosen, stimulation intensity should be set at the lowest amplitude that provides optimal benefit without persistent side effects. Though many stimulation-related adverse effects are evident immediately during the programming session, some adverse effects may be delayed in their occurrence. Especially in patients with PD, dyskinesia, hypophonia, and mood changes may emerge hours or even days after the patient has left the clinic following a DBS programming session. Because of the possibility of delayed dyskinesia, some clinicians will initiate stimulation at low, suboptimal intensity – with subsequent gradual escalation to levels ultimately producing optimal therapeutic benefit – to avoid this situation. We prefer to initiate stimulation at optimal therapeutic intensity and instruct the patient about

what to do if delayed dyskinesia or other side effects occur (see below).

Attend to final steps

Once all parameters are set, two more steps need to be undertaken. First, therapy measurements (impedance and associated current or voltage readings) at the therapeutic parameters should be documented, as well as the battery status (voltage output of the battery). Second, the clinician should clear the therapy usage counter of the neurostimulator (this occurs automatically in some device models at the end of a programming session). Clearing the counter begins a new measurement of therapy usage, allowing the clinician on the next visit to know the percentage of time and number of hours that the neurostimulator has been on. This allows the clinician to verify that DBS therapy has been administered appropriately (usually continuously for PD and dystonia and during waking hours for tremor disorders) and that the neurostimulator has not been turned off (either deliberately or inadvertently).

Patient education
Patient programmer

Being treated with DBS is a major event that can be associated with anticipation and varying levels of anxiety. It is important for patients to understand that when stimulation is turned off, their condition is the same as before surgery and symptoms will respond the same way to medications as preoperatively.

> Education about how to use their handheld patient programmer should therefore occur at the first visit, as this will greatly reduce anxiety by giving patients a sense of control.

Understandably, when patients experience new or changing symptoms they may readily attribute these to DBS. By being able to turn off their stimulator(s) they can assess whether that assumption is correct. Patients should be taught that the left neurostimulation system provides effects on the right side of the body and vice versa, so that they can appropriately assess lateralized effects. The patient's ability to turn off stimulation is valuable for those patients with PD who develop exacerbation of dyskinesia from the combination of dopaminergic medication and stimulation. In cases of significant dyskinesia, patients can be instructed to turn off stimulation until dyskinesia resolves, take a lower dose of levodopa, and then turn stimulation back on. If dyskinesia recurs, the next dose of medication can then be further reduced. In most instances this strategy will successfully reduce dyskinesia severity. Only in rare cases will it be necessary for the patient to return to the clinic to have DBS intensity turned down.

Safety

> Patients should be reminded about medical procedures that are contraindicated with the present types of DBS hardware, including many types of MRI and diathermy (the therapeutic generation of local heat in body tissues by high-frequency electromagnetic radiation, electric currents, or ultrasonic waves).

They should also be aware that certain medical tests (for example, electrocardiography and electromyography) may require that they temporarily shut off stimulation in order to eliminate artifact from the recordings. It may be helpful to summarize some of these issues in a handout that patients can share with other health professionals. For instance, when patients are scheduled for surgery, the surgeon may need guidelines for cauterization. Lastly, patients should be aware that strong magnetic fields in the environment can occasionally shut off neurostimulators that contain magnetic reed switches.

Follow-up visits (Table 5.2)

Preparation
Timing

> Following the initial programming session, patients routinely return to the clinic on a monthly basis for the first several months, followed by quarterly visits – though the schedule should be individualized to meet each patient's needs.

For example, if a stimulator adjustment caused troublesome side effects, patients should be encouraged to return sooner, whereas if they are doing well they may not need to be seen on a frequent basis.

Table 5.2 Follow-up programming checklist

Before programming

- Take interval history
  - Side effects from stimulation
  - Benefits from stimulation
  - Current medications
- Perform physical exam
  - Skin incisions
  - Neurological exam

Programming

- Record starting parameters
  - Electrode configuration, amplitude, pulse width, rate
  - Therapy impedance, current drain or current/voltage output, battery status
  - Percent use (then reset counters)
- Assess efficacy
  - If improved, but suboptimal
    - increase amplitude
    - increase pulse width or rate
  - If not improved
    - re-configure or add electrodes
  - If limited by stimulation-induced adverse effects
    - try bipolar electrode configuration
  - Document DBS settings evaluated
- Record ending parameters

After programming

- Adjust medications
- Reinforce education
  - Patient programmer use
  - Safety issues
  - Follow-up plan

Duration

Follow-up programming sessions vary in duration from 10 minutes to 1 hour, depending on the complexity of the patient, the extent of DBS reprogramming required, and any other medical

53

issues that need to be addressed. At a minimum, when a patient treated with DBS returns for a follow-up visit, it is useful to assess stimulation status, battery function, and device function, even if no reprogramming of stimulation parameters is needed.

Medication state

In contrast to the initial programming visit, follow-up visits for patients with PD do not necessarily need to occur in the off-medication state. If troublesome dyskinesia that has not improved with medication adjustment is the chief complaint, then the patient should arrive for their appointment in the "on" state, with dyskinesia present. On the other hand, if recurrent parkinsonism is the reason for the visit, patients should arrive in the "off" state after holding one or two doses of their usual scheduled medications. Patients with ET or dystonia should take their usual medications.

What to bring

For the first few follow-up visits, patients again are instructed to bring their patient programmers to reinforce proper use. Importantly, they should also bring their current medication schedule, since medication requirements likely will have changed. Some clinicians use diaries to follow patients' progress, as well (Appendix A).

Systematic approach

Interval history

Patients should be questioned about the presence, duration, and severity of motor symptoms and level of function since the last visit. The clinician should also question the patient about the presence of potential stimulation-related adverse effects, such as change in mood or behavior, speech, and visual function.

Physical exam

As infection in the region of device components can occur in a delayed manner and because erosion of skin overlying the hardware can occur after initial healing, in some cases even years later, care should be taken to examine the skin periodically.

Programming
Documenting starting parameters

Before any changes are made, the clinician should document the settings in effect at the start of the visit, as well as the therapy measurements, the percent of time that stimulation has been on, the battery status, and whether the neurostimulator is, in fact, currently on.

Impedance

A significant change in impedance relative to a previous visit combined with a complaint of reduced stimulation efficacy can alert the clinician to potential malfunction of a DBS system component, such as a fractured wire or other breach in the integrity of the DBS system.

Usage data

Anomalies of usage (such as a disparity in use between the right and left neurostimulators when two single-channel devices are present or use less than the amount to be expected) should alert the clinician to inadvertent discontinuation of stimulation and the need for troubleshooting, rather than parameter reprogramming.

Battery status

Battery longevity varies, depending on the configuration and parameters for stimulation, device use, and model of neurostimulator. Patients should be taught to use their patient programmer to check the battery status on a routine basis, but especially during periods when they are nearing the anticipated end of battery service. Clinicians should refer to the literature included with the device about battery characteristics and the point at which elective neurostimulator replacement is recommended.

Electrode selection

If care was taken to explore each electrode at the initial visit and base electrode selection on clear evidence of efficacy, then follow-up visits will usually not require a substantial change in the active electrode(s) used for stimulation. Instead, changes in the parameters of stimulation can be explored.

Amplitude selection

If some efficacy has occurred but more is needed, the amplitude is gradually increased until the desired benefit occurs.

Final steps

At the end of each programming session, the clinician will document the final stimulation parameters and therapy measurements. If not done earlier in the session, the neurostimulator usage counter should be cleared in order to reliably track therapy usage moving forward.

Patient education

At each follow-up visit, it is helpful to review the use of the patient programmer and to review safety guidelines.

Further reading

Montgomery E, Jr. Deep brain stimulation programming. In Bakay RAE, ed. *Movement Disorder Surgery: The Essentials*. New York: Thieme; 2009:187–213.

Volkmann J, Herzog J, Kopper F, Deuschl G. Introduction to the programming of deep brain stimulators. *Mov Disord* 2002;**17**(Suppl 3):S181–7.

Volkmann J, Moro E, Pahwa R. Basic algorithms for the programming of deep brain stimulation in Parkinson's disease. *Mov Disord* 2006;**21**(Suppl 14):S284–9.

Chapter 6

Managing essential tremor patients treated with deep brain stimulation

Rajesh Pahwa and Kelly E. Lyons

Tremor is one of the most common movement disorders. Among the various tremor disorders, essential tremor (ET) is the most common, affecting an estimated 10,000,000 persons in the United States.[1] There are several medical treatment options for ET, the most common including propranolol and other beta-adrenergic blockers; primidone and other anticonvulsants, such as topiramate and gabapentin; and benzodiazepines.[2] These medications, however, do not provide sufficient tremor control in up to 50% of ET patients. In these patients, deep brain stimulation (DBS) of the ventral intermediate nucleus of the thalamus (Vim) may be an appropriate treatment alternative. In the United States, Vim DBS is approved only for ET and parkinsonian tremor, but patients with a number of other tremor disorders, such as those related to multiple sclerosis and traumatic injury, have also undergone treatment with Vim DBS with varying results.[1]

> Vim thalamic DBS is most commonly used in patients with medication-resistant ET who have significant disability caused by their tremor. With appropriate DBS lead location and optimal postoperative management, there is often complete or nearly complete resolution of contralateral hand tremor.

Formal evaluations using tremor rating scales report significant improvements in hand tremor,[1,3–9] and in some cases also in head and voice tremor,[4,6–8,10] especially with bilateral procedures (Table 6.1). As with any form of therapy, the goal of DBS is to provide the maximum benefit with minimal to no adverse effects. To obtain the best outcomes, there should be appropriate patient selection, accurate lead placement, optimal programming, management of adverse effects related to stimulation and medications, and patient education. This chapter will discuss the evaluation for and management of Vim DBS in the ET patient.

Patient evaluation before beginning programming

Management begins with evaluation before DBS surgery. Prior to surgery, it is important to assess the patient to evaluate the cause, distribution, and type of the tremor and the disabilities related to tremor, such as impairment of writing, feeding, and performance of other activities. The use of formal tremor evaluation scales, such as the Fahn–Tolosa–Marin Tremor Rating Scale (TRS) (Appendix M),[11] prior to surgery will help with the long-term management of the patient by establishing the baseline severity of tremor. The TRS has three sections focusing on the severity, location, and type (rest, action, postural) of tremor; handwriting, drawing, and pouring from cups; and functional disability due to tremor. Assessment before and after surgery with an instrument such as the TRS provides a measure of change, not only immediately after surgery and during DBS programming, but also throughout post-surgical management. It is also important to document the tasks that are of particular importance to the patient, such as writing, putting on make-up, eating, holding a cup, playing a musical instrument, etc., so that performance of these particular tasks can be mimicked and targeted during device programming.

Table 6.1 Tremor improvement compared to baseline after thalamic deep brain stimulation for the treatment of essential tremor

Study	n (u/b)	Age (yrs)	Follow up (months)	Hand tremor	ADLs	Head	Voice	Stimulation settings (amplitude V; frequency Hz; pulse width µs) #		
Koller et al. 1997[3]	29/0	67	12	~60%	NR	NR	NR	3.0	153	86
Koller et al. 1999[10]	20/0	72	12	NR	NR	50%	NR	3.1	158	67
Limousin et al. 1999[4]	28/9	63	12	>75%	80%	15% (u); 85% (b)	33% (u); 40% (b)	2.4	164	84
Koller et al. 2001[5]	25/0	72	22–69	78%	NR	NR	NR	3.6	161	100
Sydow et al. 2003[6]	12/7	62	80	50–70%	39%	45% (u); 85% (b)	25% (u); 60% (b)	2.6	173	89
Putzke et al. 2004[7]	29/23	72	3–36	>83%	>63%	15–51% (u); 39–79% (b)*	15–51% (u); 39–79% (b)*	3.0	171	88
Putzke et al. 2005[8]	0/22	70	29	80–91%	69–86%	90–100%	65–100%	2.8 2.4	168 159	97 97
Pahwa et al. 2006[9]	15/7	71	60	75% (u); 65–86% (b)	51% (u); 36% (b)	NR	NR	3.6 3.6 3.2	158 155 153	111 111 129

Notes: ADLs, activities of daily living; b, bilateral; NR, not reported; u, unilateral; * reported as midline tremor; # settings at last follow up; for bilateral cases some studies reported first and second side separately while others reported the mean of all implanted leads.

Prior to initiating programming, it is helpful to obtain surgical records and review the following information.

Confirmation of lead location: Lead location, as confirmed by post-implant imaging, is helpful in determining what electrodes on the DBS lead to use for stimulation. It is also important for troubleshooting in the event that satisfactory benefit is not obtained.

Intraoperative DBS lead test stimulation: Intraoperatively, the benefits and adverse effects of various stimulation settings are tested to help confirm proper placement of the DBS lead. Particularly in the ET patient, one expects to see evidence for tremor suppression with intraoperative test stimulation and also appropriate stimulation thresholds for the induction of stimulation-related adverse effects (commonly, dysarthria and paresthesia). Intraoperative stimulation results will provide a rough guide to the clinician

in determining the most effective settings with the fewest side effects.

> However, it is important for the clinician to complete an independent screening of each electrode (see Chapter 5) to confirm the electrode configuration and parameter settings with the greatest benefit and fewest side effects. Simply adopting the intraoperative programming settings is unlikely to provide optimal effects, since the acute operative setting (both physiologically and practically) does not fully replicate the chronic state of the patient.

DBS hardware details: It is helpful for the clinician to understand which brain lead model and neurostimulator have been implanted, since each model has different specifications.

Surgical and postoperative complications: Information about any surgical or post-surgical complications should be obtained by the clinician, as well as any other information from the surgical team that may impact programming.

Patient programming

The majority of DBS clinicians initiate programming two to four weeks after Vim DBS lead implantation. This allows the brain to recover from surgery and any edema or "microlesion" effect to resolve. Since stimulation requirements for optimal tremor control tend to change during the initial weeks following DBS lead implantation, earlier programming might result in the need for more frequent or additional programming to ultimately achieve best therapeutic results. Since ET patients undergoing DBS have not received adequate tremor control with medication, many clinicians do not feel it is necessary for the patient to hold their anti-tremor medications on the day of DBS programming. As with any neurological evaluation, the patient should be assessed with a history and examination before initiating programming. Information should be collected regarding any changes in tremor since surgery and any possible complications, such as indicators of infection. The surgical site should be inspected for any redness, swelling, discharge, or excessive tenderness, and the examiner should palpate along the extension and neurostimulator to check for any abnormalities. Finally, baseline tremor should be evaluated prior to activation of stimulation. Optimally this is accomplished by using a formal rating scale, such as the TRS, but at minimum tremor should be evaluated in various body parts and functional ability assessed. This assessment usually consists of obtaining handwriting samples, performing tasks such as drinking or pouring from a cup, or mimicking tasks or movements particularly important and impaired for that specific patient. Ideally, measurements after surgery should mirror those performed prior to surgery to evaluate any changes prior to programming and throughout the programming session.

> Although ET patients may have tremor in various body parts, hand tremor is generally the most common and the most disabling, and therefore the focus of DBS programming.

The effects of stimulation depend on the location of the active electrode(s) on the DBS lead used for stimulation, stimulation parameters, and type of neural tissue that is being stimulated (axons or cell bodies). Amplitude controls the intensity or strength of the stimulation and is the most commonly adjusted parameter for Vim DBS in ET. The most common amplitude settings for Vim DBS in ET are between 1.0 and 4.0 V (with constant voltage neurostimulators). Increased amplitude results in increased spread of stimulation. Pulse width contributes to total charge density. Increasing pulse width generally allows for a reduction in amplitude, though the parameters do not exert identical clinical effects and it is important to explore different amplitude/pulse width combinations to achieve the most desirable tremor control. The most common pulse widths for Vim DBS in ET range from 60–120 μs. Rate, the number of stimulation pulses per second, is commonly set to between 130 and 185 Hz. Perhaps more so for tremor than other motor signs and symptoms, different rates of stimulation can produce greater or lesser levels of symptom control. Though not typically the major parameter adjusted to control tremor, rate can be altered to explore effects on optimizing tremor control when other parameter adjustments have been completed.

Prior to initiating DBS programming, electrode impedance measurements should be performed to confirm integrity of the DBS system and its connections and also to document a baseline measurement for future reference during troubleshooting.

The next step includes assessing the efficacy and adverse effects of stimulation by screening each individual electrode on the DBS lead. This is performed in the monopolar mode by assigning one of the electrodes to have negative polarity and designating the neurostimulator case to be positive. The initial stimulation parameters typically start at amplitude 0 V, pulse width 60 or 90 μs, and frequency of 130–145 Hz. Stimulation amplitude is gradually increased (by about 0.5 V every few seconds), and all other parameters kept constant. The patient is observed for benefit and adverse effects, such as dysarthria and paresthesia. For each individual electrode, the threshold amplitude for benefit and the development of adverse effects should be determined. The type, location, and degree of benefit as well as the type, location, and severity of adverse effects should be noted. The amplitude is increased until adverse effects are persistent and uncomfortable. The presence of persistent stimulation-induced adverse effects at a low amplitude of stimulation (less than 2.0 V) suggests that the electrode is not optimally placed. For example, persistent paresthesia occurring at a low amplitude of stimulation suggests that the electrode is too posterior and is stimulating the ventralis caudalis nucleus of the thalamus (the part of the thalamus mediating sensation), tonic contraction of the face or limb at low levels of stimulation suggests that the electrode is too lateral and is stimulating the internal capsule, and stimulation-related dizziness at a low level of stimulation suggests that the electrode is too deep.

> The results of the electrode screening provide the basis for selecting the best electrode to use for monopolar stimulation. The electrode that provides the best tremor control with the fewest adverse effects is chosen as the possible electrode for final use.

The amplitude used is that required to achieve complete tremor suppression and is ideally 0.5–1.0 V below the threshold for development of adverse effects to ensure a sufficient therapeutic window.

> If complete tremor suppression is not achieved using monopolar stimulation with a single electrode but stimulation is well tolerated, an electrode configuration employing two (or rarely, even three) electrodes assigned to have negative polarity is tried to determine the configuration providing optimal effects.

> If achieving optimal tremor control is hampered by the occurrence of stimulation-induced adverse effects, then stimulation using a bipolar electrode configuration should be attempted, since this provides a more constricted field of stimulation and may consequently reduce adverse effects by limiting electrical current spread to adjacent brain structures.

The electrode that provided the best tremor control via monopolar stimulation during the screening process is chosen as the negative electrode for bipolar stimulation. An adjacent electrode on either side is then set to be the positive electrode. As with monopolar stimulation, the threshold for efficacy and adverse effects is determined for relevant bipolar configurations. Switching the polarity of the selected electrodes might sometimes improve efficacy and provide the best tremor control. For example, if it is determined that the best electrode for tremor control is electrode 2 during monopolar screening, then electrodes 2 and 1 might be assessed in a bipolar configuration. Initially, electrode 2 would be negative and electrode 1 positive. However, the polarity may be reversed, such that electrode 2 is positive and electrode 1 negative. Other derivative bipolar configurations can then be explored if necessary.

> If satisfactory tremor suppression without adverse effects is still not achieved, the pulse width and then the frequency should be increased in an effort to achieve better tremor control.

For bilateral implants, the screening process should be completed for each side individually and further adjustments then made after both leads are delivering stimulation. An algorithm for programming an ET patient after Vim DBS is shown in Figure 6.1.

Typical, final settings for Vim stimulation are an amplitude of 1–4 V, a pulse width of 60–120 µs, and a rate of 130–185 Hz. For one of the commonly used neurostimulators used for ET patients (Soletra, Medtronic, Inc.), an amplitude higher than 3.6 V used for chronic stimulation results in accelerated drain on the battery; thus, to maximize battery life, if an amplitude greater than 3.6 V is needed for optimal tremor control, a lower amplitude should be explored in conjunction with an increased pulse width or rate. Once the best combination of parameters is identified that provides the best efficacy with the fewest adverse effects, the patient is sent home on those settings and the details recorded in the medical chart.

Stimulation-related adverse effects

Stimulation-related adverse effects at levels of stimulation needed for tremor control usually occur due to suboptimal DBS lead location or failure to select the most optimally located electrode on the DBS lead for stimulation. Stimulation-related adverse effects for DBS in the region of the Vim include paresthesia, dysarthria, incoordination, pain, asthenia, abnormal thinking, and headache.[7,9]

Tremor medication adjustments

If patients are treated with unilateral Vim stimulation, anti-tremor medications are usually maintained, if tolerated, to help treat tremor on the other side of

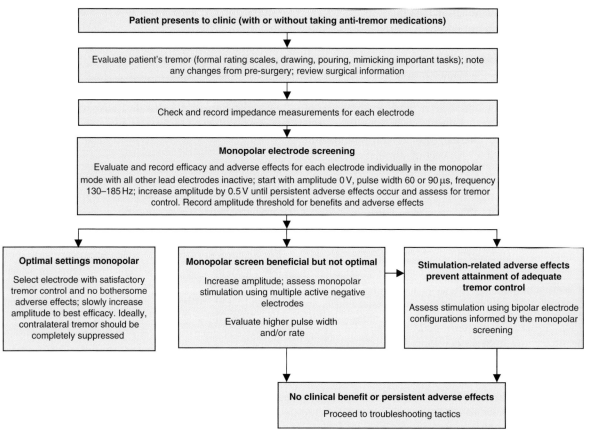

Figure 6.1 Programming algorithm for ventral intermedius deep brain stimulation (Vim DBS) in essential tremor patients.

the body. If the patient is treated with bilateral Vim DBS or if the tremor on the opposite side is not disabling, anti-tremor medications should be gradually tapered and discontinued.

Follow up

Once optimal settings are determined, patients are seen every 6–12 months for evaluation and minor adjustments, if necessary. Often, stimulation parameters remain remarkably stable over time and provide excellent tremor suppression for many years.

In a minority of cases, efficacy may wane over time, usually because the DBS lead location is not ideal. Some loss of tremor control can occur due to disease progression; however, this can often be corrected by a gradual increase in the amplitude of stimulation or addition of an extra active electrode.

Patient instructions

The neurostimulator can be turned off by the patient using the patient programmer.

To prolong neurostimulator battery longevity, patients are usually instructed to turn the device off at night, since their tremor will cease with sleep and respond quickly the following morning when the device is turned back on. In patients with bilateral treatment, if significant speech or gait abnormalities occur with both stimulators on, consider having the patient keep one side of stimulation off when speaking or walking to eliminate these adverse effects and both sides on while they are seated and working with both hands.

Management of other forms of tremor

Although Vim DBS is approved in the United States by the Food and Drug Administration only to treat tremor caused by ET and Parkinson's disease, it has been used in an attempt to control other forms of tremor, such as that associated with multiple sclerosis and traumatic brain injury.[1] In general, the postoperative management of these other forms of tremor is similar to that described for ET.

References

1. Lyons KE, Pahwa R. Deep brain stimulation and tremor. *Neurotherapeutics* 2008;5(2):331–8.

2. Zesiewicz TA, Elble R, Louis ED, et al. Practice parameter: therapies for essential tremor: report of the Quality Standards Subcommittee of the American Academy of Neurology. *Neurology* 2005;**64** (12):2008–20.

3. Koller W, Pahwa R, Busenbark K, et al. High-frequency unilateral thalamic stimulation in the treatment of essential and parkinsonian tremor. *Ann Neurol* 1997;**42** (3):292–9.

4. Limousin P, Speelman JD, Gielen F, Janssens M. Multicentre European study of thalamic stimulation in parkinsonian and essential tremor. *J Neurol Neurosurg Psychiatry* 1999;**66**(3):289–96.

5. Koller WC, Lyons KE, Wilkinson SB, Troster AI, Pahwa R. Long-term safety and efficacy of unilateral deep brain stimulation of the thalamus in essential tremor. *Mov Disord* 2001;**16**(3):464–8.

6. Sydow O, Thobois S, Alesch F, Speelman JD. Multicentre European study of thalamic stimulation in essential tremor: a six year follow up. *J Neurol Neurosurg Psychiatry* 2003;**74**(10):1387–91.

7. Putzke JD, Wharen RE, Jr., Obwegeser AA, et al. Thalamic deep brain stimulation for essential tremor: recommendations for long-term outcome analysis. *Can J Neurol Sci* 2004;**31**(3):333–42.

8. Putzke JD, Uitti RJ, Obwegeser AA, Wszolek ZK, Wharen RE. Bilateral thalamic deep brain stimulation: midline tremor control. *J Neurol Neurosurg Psychiatry* 2005;**76**(5):684–90.

9. Pahwa R, Lyons KE, Wilkinson SB, et al. Long-term evaluation of deep brain stimulation of the thalamus. *J Neurosurg* 2006;**104**(4):506–12.

10. Koller WC, Lyons KE, Wilkinson SB, Pahwa R. Efficacy of unilateral deep brain stimulation of the VIM nucleus of the thalamus for essential head tremor. *Mov Disord* 1999;**14**(5):847–50.

11. Fahn S, Tolosa E, Marin C. Clinical rating scale for tremor. In Jankovic J, Tolosa E, eds. *Parkinson's Disease and Movement Disorders*. Munich: Urban & Schwarzenberg; 1988:225–34.

Managing Parkinson's disease patients treated with deep brain stimulation

Rajeev Kumar and Lindsey Johnson

Introduction

Deep brain stimulation (DBS) has become a widely used treatment for medication-refractory movement disorders, including Parkinson's disease (PD), dystonia, and various forms of tremor. For PD, DBS has been applied to the ventral intermedius (Vim) nucleus of the thalamus, globus pallidus internus (GPi), subthalamic nucleus (STN), and pedunculopontine nucleus (PPN). The exact mechanism of action of DBS is unknown but is consistent with high frequency stimulation blocking the activity of the target nucleus and other regions to which there are connections by direct or indirect means. Some have speculated that the mechanism of action of DBS is consistent with a "jamming of the neuronal message transmitted through the stimulated structure and desynchronization of abnormal oscillations."[1,2]

Vim DBS has been shown to markedly improve tremor in a fashion similar to that achieved with thalamotomy but with fewer persistent adverse effects.[1,3] Although Vim DBS can markedly improve parkinsonian tremor, this form of therapy does not significantly improve other features of parkinsonism.[1,3,4] However, GPi DBS and STN DBS can markedly improve all levodopa-responsive motor features of parkinsonism.[1,5–8] PPN DBS is a new, experimental target that is being investigated for treatment of refractory parkinsonian gait and balance disorders. Preliminary results suggest that this may be a promising therapy.[11–15] A few groups have also presented limited data suggesting that stimulation of the zona incerta (Zi) region may be beneficial.[16,17]

We describe our practical approach to postoperative patient management, including adjusting stimulation parameters, altering pharmacological therapy, and identifying complications. We propose guidelines based on our clinical experience and that of other groups. We recognize that alternative, equally valid approaches may exist.

The practical matter of programming DBS settings in PD patients with DBS leads implanted in the GPi, STN, or PPN is more complex than thalamic Vim DBS for tremor, and obtaining optimal results can be a time-consuming process. In addition, adjustments in stimulation parameters must often be accompanied by alterations in anti-parkinsonian medication in order to improve both motor fluctuations and levodopa-induced dyskinesia. Patients and their caregivers must be able to effectively participate in frequent follow-up visits for evaluations and stimulator adjustments and have realistic expectations of the improvement in motor function and quality of life that DBS can provide.

Patients with PD undergoing GPi or STN DBS typically have disabling medication-refractory motor fluctuation, often with levodopa-induced dyskinesia, despite maximized pharmacological therapy, or have significant medication intolerance that makes pharmacological management unsatisfactory. As discussed in Chapter 2, use of DBS is generally restricted to patients without significant cognitive impairment. Our experience suggests that elderly patients predisposed to cognitive impairment may experience cognitive worsening, especially with bilateral STN surgery[18]; therefore, we routinely refer all patients for preoperative detailed neuropsychological testing to assess whether patients have the cognitive reserves to withstand surgery.[19,20] Patients must be motivated and be able to actively participate during an awake surgery that may be emotionally stressful and lengthy. As a result, we commonly exclude patients from DBS implantation if they have active psychiatric symptoms, since such patients may become agitated during surgery and are commonly cognitively impaired.

Clinical effects of DBS of Vim, STN, and GPi

> The clinical effects of Vim DBS in PD are outlined in Table 7.1: patients experience virtually complete suppression of off-period contralateral tremor and mild improvement in rigidity, but no improvement in bradykinesia.[21]

However, DBS lead placement in the centromedian/parafascicularis (CM/Pf) nucleus of the thalamus or anterior to the Vim (i.e., in the region of the Voa/Vop nuclei) may suppress levodopa-induced dyskinesia.[22] Disability as measured by the Unified Parkinson's Disease Rating Scale (UPDRS) is not improved with thalamic stimulation because most disability in PD stems from bradykinesia and gait disorders. However, manual tasks worsened by tremor, such as handwriting, may be improved.

> A dramatic and beneficial effect of both GPi and STN DBS has been consistently observed. Both interventions when applied bilaterally result in significant improvements in quality of life and in motor fluctuation and dyskinesia as measured by patient home diary assessments.

In a large multicenter study, "on" time without dyskinesia during the waking day increased from 25–30% at baseline to 65–75% 6 months postoperatively, and in a complementary fashion these interventions markedly decreased "off" time and "on" time with dyskinesia.[23] Non-motor fluctuation also improves following STN DBS, with the most notable improvements in asthenia, irritability, and drenching sweats.[24] In addition, improved quality and increased total sleep time, as well as decreased daytime sleepiness (likely due to increased nocturnal mobility), have been reported.[25,26]

> The degree of improvement obtained with levodopa (usually the first morning dose of anti-parkinsonian medication with or without an additional 50–100 mg of levodopa, see Chapter 2) after overnight withdrawal of anti-parkinsonian medication is highly predictive of the response to STN DBS and probably also to GPi DBS.[27–29]

Therefore, the levodopa test is an important part of the evaluation to determine the degree of benefit obtainable with DBS.

> With the exception of tremor, signs that are not improved with levodopa usually fail to improve with DBS; these include cognitive and psychiatric problems, on-period freezing, and levodopa-refractory dysarthria, dysphagia, and postural instability.[29,30]

Furthermore, the levodopa test reinforces for the patient and family realistic expectations of the potential maximal results of surgery.

Parkinson's disease-associated camptocormia is characterized by marked flexion of the trunk and often responds poorly to pharmacological treatment. Several reports document sustained improvement of PD-associated camptocormia with bilateral GPi or STN DBS.[31–34]

Choice of stimulation location

There is ongoing controversy as to the best overall management strategy when applying DBS to a broad population of PD patients. Nevertheless, creating a customized plan for each individual patient that takes into account the patient's motor and non-motor symptoms, degree of asymmetry, and psychosocial situation seems most prudent.

> GPi and STN DBS can each be applied successfully with relatively similar beneficial effects.

GPi DBS directly suppresses dyskinesia but little medication reduction may be achieved, whereas STN DBS predominantly has an indirect anti-dyskinetic effect achieved through medication reduction. In our experience, STN DBS may also have a greater anti-tremor effect compared to GPi DBS. Unilateral GPi or STN DBS has significant beneficial effects (although substantially less than bilateral DBS) and may expose patients to less upfront risk than that of a bilateral procedure (a second stimulator may then be added when symptoms progress or if the effects of unilateral stimulation are inadequate). Unilateral STN DBS has a greater likelihood of producing mild cognitive adverse effects than unilateral GPi DBS, especially on verbal fluency.[35] Bilateral STN DBS has a greater propensity to cause a variety of behavioral adverse effects (including mania and

Table 7.1 Comparison of the clinical effects of GPi, STN, and Vim deep brain stimulation in Parkinson's disease

	GPi DBS	**STN DBS**	**Vim DBS**
Overall clinical effects of bilateral DBS	Mean improvements in rating scales: Off-period parkinsonism 30–50% On-period parkinsonism 0–25% On-period dyskinesia reduced 66–90% Off-period dystonia usually improved	Mean improvements in rating scales: Off-period parkinsonism 45–65% On-period parkinsonism 10–30% On-period dyskinesia reduced 67–83% Off-period dystonia usually improved	Tremor improvement 90% Rigidity improvement only minimal ADLs not improved overall
Overall clinical effects of unilateral DBS	Mean improvements: Off-period parkinsonism 10–35% On-period parkinsonism not improved On-period dyskinesia reduced 70–80% Off-period dystonia usually improved	Mean improvements: Off-period parkinsonism 25–30% Effects on on-period parkinsonism and dyskinesia not studied Off-period dystonia usually improved	Contralateral limb tremor improvement 90% Axial and ipsilateral tremor only minimally improved Rigidity improvement only minimal ADLs not improved overall
Microlesion effect	Minor beneficial improvement in off-period parkinsonism occurs in some patients Moderate anti-dyskinetic effect may be seen	Mild beneficial effects on off-period parkinsonism occur in some patients Effect on dyskinesia is variable (may be pro-dyskinetic in some and anti-dyskinetic in other patients)	Significant reduction in contralateral tremor measurable for up to three months in some patients; occasional patients show marked persistent tremor reduction
Regional stimulation within the nucleus	Dorsal electrodes: greater anti-parkinsonian effect and can produce contralateral stimulation-induced dyskinesia Ventral electrodes: greater anti-dyskinetic effect and can block beneficial effects of levodopa on bradykinesia and gait	Pro-dyskinetic effect often observed Behavioral or affective changes can occur with stimulation of limbic portion of STN or adjacent hypothalamus; acute stimulation-related depression can occur when using the electrode inferior to STN in SNr	None
Mechanism of effects on levodopa-induced dyskinesia	Anti-dyskinetic effect of microlesion and direct anti-dyskinetic effect of stimulation	Mainly due to reduction in dopaminergic drug dosage; in some patients, microlesion effect directly reduces dyskinesia (possibly due to lesion of lenticular fasciculus) STN stimulation commonly has a pro-dyskinetic effect	Stimulation using electrodes placed within or adjacent to CM/Pf or Voa/Vop may suppress contralateral dyskinesia

Table 7.1 (*cont.*)

	GPi DBS	STN DBS	Vim DBS
		Stimulation above the STN in the zona incerta or below the STN in the SNr may directly suppress dyskinesia in a manner similar to GPi DBS	
Stimulation-induced dyskinesia	Onset within one to two minutes	Onset usually within minutes, but occasionally delayed up to days with chronic stimulation; tends to improve with time	None
	Contralateral	Contralateral or even ipsilateral	Ventral spread of stimulation to the cerebellothalamic fibers may result in stimulation-induced ataxia
	Similar form and distribution to the patient's preoperative peak dose levodopa-induced dyskinesia (though usually milder); usually abates in minutes or hours with chronic stimulation	Two different forms: Hemiballistic/ hemichoreic and sometimes very different from the patient's preoperative peak-dose levodopa-induced dyskinesia, or Dyskinesia resembling the patient's preoperative peak dose dyskinesia Both types may occur in the same individual; type 1 at low amplitude stimulation and type 2 at high amplitude stimulation Levodopa and STN DBS have a synergistic effect in promoting dyskinesia; therefore, drug reduction is necessary to reduce dyskinesia and allow the use of higher stimulation parameters	Rebound tremor may occur with discontinuation of stimulation
Postoperative medication management	Usually no change required, though some patients are able to reduce medication; patients with severe preoperative dyskinesia may tolerate higher doses of medication following DBS	Mean reduction in medication dosage 50% (range 0–100%)	Usually no change. Occasional patients with severe tremor and very mild bradykinesia may be able to reduce anti-parkinsonian medication
Timing of anti-parkinsonian effects	Tremor improvement almost immediate Most other features of parkinsonism improve within one minute, but full benefit may take minutes to hours to days	Tremor improvement almost immediate Most other features of parkinsonism improve within one minute, but full benefit may take minutes to hours to days	Tremor improvement almost immediate

Table 7.1 (cont.)

	GPi DBS	STN DBS	Vim DBS
Major stimulation-induced adverse effects due to spread of stimulation to adjacent structures	Ventrally to optic tract: phosphenes, nausea Posteriorly or medially to internal capsule: tonic muscle contraction	Anterolaterally to corticospinal tract: tonic contraction Posteromedially to medial lemniscus: paresthesia Inferomedially to oculomotor nucleus or its fascicles: diplopia	Ventrally to cerebellothalamic fibers: ataxia Laterally to internal capsule: tonic contraction Posteriorly to primary thalamic somatosensory nucleus (Vc): paresthesia

Notes: ADL, activities of daily living; CM/Pf, centromedian/ parafascicularis; DBS, deep brain stimulation; GPi, globus pallidus internus; SNr, substantia nigra reticulate; STN, subthalamic nucleus; Vim, ventral intermedius.

depression) not usually seen with GPi DBS, especially in patients with pre-existing psychiatric problems. As a result, GPi DBS might be a better target in patients thought to have a greater chance of psychiatric or cognitive worsening with DBS surgery. STN DBS may also be appropriate in selected patients who are unable to tolerate adequate doses of anti-parkinsonian medication (because of somnolence, severe gastrointestinal adverse effects, or psychiatric adverse effects in the absence of cognitive impairment), since this treatment typically treats cardinal motor symptoms without the need for high levels of anti-parkinsonian medication.[36] Some clinicians even report that up to 10% of all patients treated with bilateral STN DBS are able to stop all drug therapy at 1–2 years postoperatively, at least for some period of time.[9] Marked benefit on co-morbid obsessive-compulsive disorder (OCD) in PD patients has also been achieved with bilateral STN DBS,[37,38] and marked reduction in dopaminergic therapy with STN DBS has allowed resolution of drug-induced impulse-control disorders.[39,40] Furthermore, STN DBS often leads to longer neurostimulator battery longevity compared to GPi DBS due to the lower stimulation parameters typically required.[41,42] This results in fewer surgeries in order to replace a primary cell neurostimulator and, as a result, less cost. The STN may be an easier surgical target because it is more clearly identified by MRI. Despite these advantages compared with GPi DBS, STN DBS may require more frequent follow-up visits, with complex postoperative management of medication and stimulation-induced adverse effects sometimes required.[42]

We and others have found that optimally applying unilateral STN DBS in many PD patients may be difficult because of the need to reduce anti-parkinsonian medication in order to reduce dyskinesia on the side of the body contralateral to stimulation. This medication reduction may result in relative under treatment and worsening of parkinsonism on the side of the body ipsilateral to stimulation. On the other hand, we have had excellent results and no difficulty with medication management using unilateral STN DBS in patients with highly asymmetrical, medication-refractory, tremor-dominant PD.

Preoperative patient management

In patients with PD, interventions that maximize off-period parkinsonism and reduce the chance of intraoperative confusion may be valuable, since they may facilitate detection of improvement in parkinsonian signs during intraoperative DBS test stimulation and improve the validity of patient-reported adverse effects. Preoperative reduction in anti-parkinsonian medication can achieve both these goals.

> Therefore, we usually withhold levodopa and catechol-O-methyltransferase (COMT) inhibitors for 12 hours prior to surgery and during surgery.

If patients are on high doses of dopamine agonists, it is often helpful to discontinue these 24–48 hours before surgery because of their long half life. Some clinicians prefer to reduce dopamine agonists one month or more prior to STN DBS surgery to eliminate the effects of these drugs completely. Lastly, other anti-parkinsonian medications that have a greater tendency to cause confusion, such as anticholinergics and amantadine, may be tapered prior to surgery to eliminate their contribution to adverse cognitive effects.

General postoperative patient management issues

Postoperative issues

Elderly patients sometimes develop postoperative confusion following bilateral DBS lead implantation that may last from a day to a few weeks. In general, only supportive therapy is required, and anti-parkinsonian medication can usually be reinstituted during this period – though typically at a reduced dose compared to preoperatively. In rare cases of prolonged confusion accompanied by psychotic features (such as hallucinations), the use of atypical antipsychotic agents, such as clozapine, may be useful. Postoperative confusion has been reported less frequently with GPi lead implantation compared to STN surgery, suggesting that this adverse effect might be somewhat specific to STN surgery rather than entirely being a non-specific effect caused by anti-parkinsonian drug withdrawal and the demands of surgery. If the patient is lucid postoperatively, no change in drug dosage is immediately necessary. As noted above, many patients with GPi lead implantation will note improvement in both off-period parkinsonism and dyskinesia as a result of the micro-pallidotomy effect.

> STN lead implantation may reduce dyskinesia, possibly due to micro-lesioning of the pallidal outflow fibers (especially the lenticular fasciculus), or more commonly may improve off-period parkinsonism and reduce the threshold for anti-parkinsonian medication to induce dyskinesia (probably as a result of micro-lesioning of the STN itself). In the latter case, it is often necessary to temporarily reduce anti-parkinsonian medication in order to reduce dyskinesia.

Mild chorea may occasionally occur following STN lead implantation. Generally this subsides within 48 hours; however, in our experience, this may rarely take 1–2 months to resolve. If significant chorea is present, a temporary reduction in levodopa dosage by 50% or more is prudent until the chorea resolves.

Where concern exists about the location of the implanted lead because of inadequate response to intraoperative stimulation or other technical factors, externalization of the DBS lead via a percutaneous extension may be advisable for a period of test stimulation using an external neurostimulator. If acceptable results were obtained from intraoperative electrophysiological mapping and test stimulation of the DBS lead, then no period of test stimulation via a percutaneously externalized lead is necessary prior to implantation of the implantable neurostimulator(s).

We usually allow patients to recover from surgery for one to two weeks prior to beginning DBS device programming. This allows wounds to heal and some of the more obvious micro-lesion effects to subside (presumably as peri-lesional edema subsides).

The total effect of DBS is achieved as a result of the micro-lesion caused by lead implantation (minor effect) and the direct effect of stimulation (major effect). Commonly, the benefit achieved with micro-lesioning is maximal immediately postoperatively and declines over several weeks as the edema surrounding the implanted lead resolves. Nevertheless, some microlesion effects may be noticeable for at least six months.[18,43]

The role of postoperative CT and MRI scanning

Postoperative CT or MRI scans can be used to determine if the DBS leads have been implanted in an optimal location and to exclude hemorrhage and other surgical complications.[44] We routinely perform postoperative stereotactic CT scans with 1 mm slice thickness, and in select cases postoperative MRI. We have found that DBS lead electrode localization based on imaging can be a helpful tool in selecting the electrodes that are most likely to be efficacious for STN or GPi stimulation.[45,46]

> In our experience, electrodes located in the dorsolateral portion of the STN are usually most beneficial (in contrast with some reports suggesting that stimulation above the STN is optimal). Similarly, electrodes located in the center of the GPi are most commonly selected for chronic stimulation.

Postoperative imaging is also extremely useful when patients have received suboptimal clinical benefit from DBS to document DBS lead location and to assess the need for lead repositioning.

Software-based image fusion of a postoperative CT or MRI scan with a preoperative MRI scan provides data regarding exact lead location.[46,47] The clarity of the postoperative image of each electrode on the DBS lead can be improved by adjusting the window settings to reduce the artifact. The location of each electrode can be plotted, based on the image and the knowledge of the electrode spacing on the lead. The position of each electrode can be assessed on the co-registered preoperative MRI with respect to being inside or outside of the anatomical target, and the distance from the ideal location based on the preoperative surgical plan.

MRI may lead to device movement, heating, program interference, and induced voltage from the electromagnetic fields used during the imaging process.[44,48] CT scans do not interact with metallic components of the DBS device.[46,47] Problems created by imaging are influenced by a number of factors, including the specific device implanted, the MRI procedure, electrical parameters of the neurostimulation system, field strength of the magnetic resonance (MR) system, orientation of the neurostimulator, type of radio frequency (RF) coil, amount of RF energy administered, and how the specific absorption rate (SAR) is calculated by the MR system.[48] The SAR is the rate of energy absorption in the body when exposed to RF. Heating of the DBS device is a very important safety issue because irreversible thermal damage is associated with $8°C+$ increase in temperature.[47] Indeed, diathermy can result in fatal electrode heating and is contraindicated with DBS.[49]

Clinicians should consult current safety guidelines published by the device manufacturer before performing any imaging study on a patient with implanted DBS leads or a DBS system.

Programming of DBS
DBS device programming in PD patients

The practical matter of programming DBS devices in PD patients with leads implanted in the GPi, STN, or PPN is more complex than programming

thalamic Vim DBS, and obtaining optimal results can be a time-consuming process. In addition, adjustments in stimulation parameters must often be accompanied by alterations in anti-parkinsonian medication in order to improve both motor fluctuation and levodopa-induced dyskinesia. Patients and their caregivers must be able to effectively participate in relatively frequent follow-up visits for evaluations and stimulator adjustments and have realistic expectations about the benefits that stimulation can provide.

The fundamentals of DBS programming are discussed in Chapter 5, and the reader is invited to review that chapter before moving on to the specific issues pertaining to programming DBS devices in PD patients that will now be discussed.

Assessment and record keeping of clinical effects of DBS in PD patients

---

Recording relatively detailed notes about the observations made during DBS programming is very helpful in allowing a systematic determination of the best stimulation settings. For each electrode configuration, it is important to record the amplitude threshold for stimulation-induced adverse effects, the nature of the adverse effects (e.g., tonic contraction due to current spread to the corticospinal tract at 4.0 V), a qualitative description of the degree of benefit (e.g., very good benefit for tremor, moderate improvement of arm bradykinesia), and perhaps a cross-reference to the UPDRS motor score.

In patients with tremor, repeated examination of a task that is highly sensitive to tremor for that particular patient, such as writing and drawing a spiral, may be necessary to differentiate between otherwise clinically similar effects achieved by different DBS electrode configurations and stimulation parameters. It may be valuable to note the severity and distribution of signs and symptoms on both sides of the body (not just contralateral to stimulation), since sometimes DBS may produce ipsilateral effects. For patients with PD, a description of the nature, severity, and distribution of off-period dystonia and on-period or stimulation-induced dyskinesia is also important.

Scheduling DBS programming sessions: Vim DBS

Patients should withhold anti-parkinsonian medication at least overnight prior to the initial programming session. Usually a concentrated period of about one hour is adequate to determine the most effective anti-tremor settings in the vast majority of patients. The algorithm (Figure 7.1) begins with assessment of stimulation-induced adverse effects for each electrode on each DBS lead, followed by evaluation of therapeutic efficacy for each electrode. Many programming clinicians, however, perform an initial evaluation of both stimulation-induced adverse effects and efficacy for each electrode in sequence.

Vim DBS programming algorithm (Figure 7.1)

1. Before beginning DBS programming it is useful to record the impedance masurements for each of the four electrodes. Being able to refer to the initial impedances and other electrical properties of the system can be helpful in troubleshooting future hardware problems.
2. If two leads have been implanted, each side should initially be programmed independently, starting with monopolar stimulation.
3. The threshold for persistent stimulation-induced adverse effects should be determined for each electrode in the monopolar mode. The recommended initial stimulation parameters for Vim DBS are amplitude 0 V, pulse width 60 or 90 μs, and frequency 130–160 Hz. The amplitude should be gradually increased by 0.5 V every 5–60 seconds (keeping other stimulation parameters constant) while constantly monitoring the patient for subjective and objective adverse effects. An abrupt increase to high amplitude may cause uncomfortable tonic muscle contraction or paresthesia, but tolerance to these adverse effects (especially paresthesia) commonly develops if the amplitude is increased slowly. The amplitude should be increased until persistent adverse effects occur, and then the clinician should note and record the threshold amplitude and nature of adverse effects.

Analyzing the threshold and nature of the adverse effects with monopolar stimulation allows one to determine the relative location of each of the electrodes to adjacent anatomical structures (Table 7.1).

Determination of efficacy on tremor

1. First perform a baseline assessment with stimulation off at the beginning of each programming session for comparison and assessment of stimulation benefits.
2. The results of monopolar stimulation provide a base of information that allows one to arrive at bipolar electrode combinations that are more likely to yield good results, if it becomes necessary to explore bipolar electrode configurations.

   (a) Using monopolar stimulation for each electrode, test the effects of stimulation on tremor at an amplitude 0.5–1.0 V below the threshold for persistent adverse effects. Record the clinical benefit noted for each electrode. The onset and offset of effect on tremor is virtually immediate, so assessments need not be significantly delayed after beginning stimulation with new parameters. If complete tremor suppression can be achieved in the target limb with monopolar stimulation, no further electrode combinations need be tested.

   (b) Repeat the above process using the other side (for bilaterally implanted patients).

3. If monopolar stimulation fails to provide adequate tremor control due to stimulation-related adverse effects, then explore logical bipolar electrode configurations based on observations from the monopolar electrode screening. Decide which one or two electrodes provides the best anti-tremor effects with monopolar stimulation, and begin bipolar stimulation by using these electrodes, determining the threshold for adverse effects and then efficacy of stimulation.
4. If complete tremor suppression is still not achieved, increase the rate, up to 185 Hz, and re-evaluate efficacy.
5. Test double monopolar stimulation using the best electrode in combination with an electrode adjacent to it using the same methodology if tremor is not completely suppressed with the single monopolar and bipolar electrode combinations. Many clinicians would explore stimulation using a double monopolar

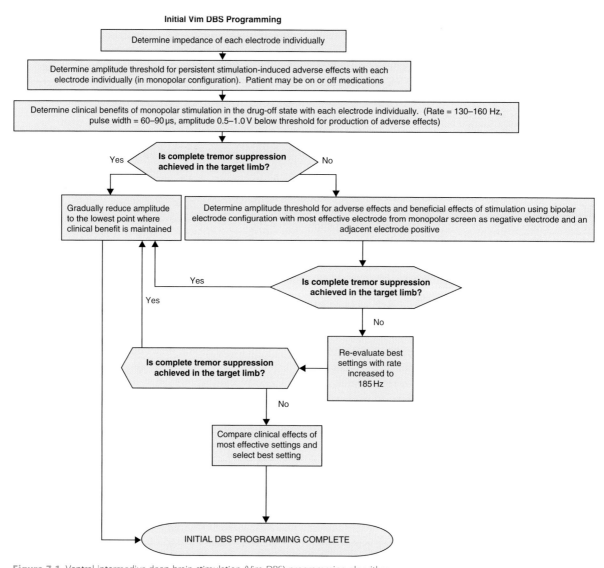

Figure 7.1 Ventral intermedius deep brain stimulation (Vim DBS) programming algorithm.

configuration before moving on to a bipolar configuration.

6. Rank in order the electrode configurations that provide the best tremor suppression for each side.
7. Once the best electrode combination has been determined, stimulation parameters can be optimized.
8. At the end of each programming session send the patient home on the optimal settings thus far determined.

Determination of efficacy on drug-induced dyskinesia in PD

In patients with PD and levodopa-induced dyskinesia, spread of stimulation current beyond the Vim to the CM/Pf or Voa/Vop regions of the thalamus may block dyskinesia. Verifying the presence or absence of this effect with the anti-tremor stimulation settings in place after levodopa administration is important, since an anti-dyskinetic effect may allow more aggressive drug therapy of off-period bradykinesia and other features of parkinsonism.

Delayed stimulation adjustment and medication adjustment

Stimulation parameters required to optimally treat motor symptoms become fairly stable by one month postoperatively, and usually only minor adjustments (such as slightly increasing the amplitude) may be necessary beyond three months. Tolerance has not been reported with Vim DBS for PD, but some patients may develop rebound increase in tremor when turning stimulation off at night.[3,21] As a result, some PD patients must keep stimulation on at night to permit sleep.

Although the majority of patients with PD undergoing Vim DBS require little or no change in medication, patients taking large doses of levodopa to suppress tremor may be able to reduce medication somewhat.[3,21]

Scheduling DBS programming sessions: GPi, STN, or PPN DBS

> Programming sessions should generally be no longer than a few hours in duration, as longer sessions often result in patient fatigue and produce variable and unreliable patient performance during tests of bradykinesia.

Most DBS programming in PD patients is performed with patients off medication, and ideally sessions should be scheduled in the morning after overnight drug withdrawal. However, in patients with extremely severe off-period immobility or lack of caregiver support, this may not be easily accomplished without hospitalization and inpatient programming. As a result, a reasonable compromise is to have patients take their first dose of levodopa in the morning to allow them to attend the clinic in a mobile drug-on state; once in the clinic, the effects of anti-parkinsonian medication may be allowed to wear off so that programming can begin in the early afternoon. Patients can then be given levodopa at the conclusion of the session if necessary to assess the effects of stimulation in conjunction with medication before they are sent home. Rare patients may become virtually anarthric and unable to communicate or too disabled to cooperate during programming when completely off medication; such patients may be given just enough anti-parkinsonian medication to induce a suboptimal "on" response without dyskinesia and allow participation. Also in such patients, greater emphasis can be placed on the response of rigidity to various DBS settings, since testing rigidity requires less active patient cooperation.[50] Assessment of the effects of DBS on drug-induced dyskinesia is often best performed in the afternoon, once patients have taken more than one dose of levodopa prior to attending the clinic, since dyskinesia commonly exhibits a diurnal pattern (mild in the morning, with worsening in the afternoon and evening).

GPi DBS programming algorithm (Figure 7.2)

Initial DBS programming

1. The principles of initial programming are identical to those used for thalamic stimulation, with initial stimulation parameters for GPi DBS being amplitude 0 V, pulse width 60 or 90 µs, and frequency 130–160 Hz.

For patients with PD undergoing GPi DBS (or STN DBS, for that matter), determination of amplitude thresholds for induction of adverse effects may be performed in the medication-on or medication-off state for all electrode combinations. Determining these adverse effect thresholds with the patient on medication can reduce the time patients need to spend off medication, as the stimulation amplitude can more quickly be increased to the previously determined threshold level when later testing stimulation efficacy in the medication-off state (see below). This is particularly useful for patients who have great difficulty tolerating being off medication for a significant length of time.

> Many clinicians simply perform assessment of both adverse effect induction and efficacy in concert with the patient in the off-medication state.

Two groups have reported on the apparent functional differences between dorsal and ventral globus pallidus stimulation (Figure 7.3).[27,51]

71

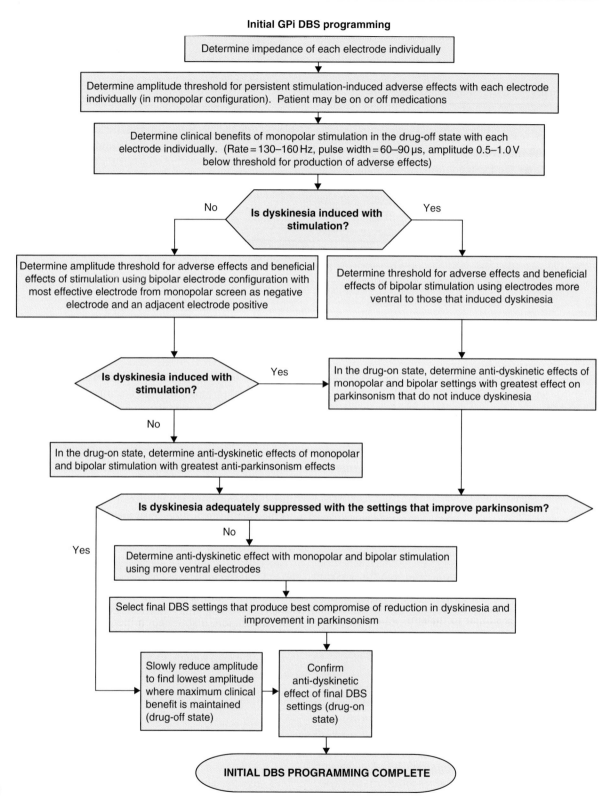

Figure 7.2 Globus pallidus internus deep brain stimulation (GPi DBS) programming algorithm.

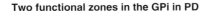

Two functional zones in the GPi in PD

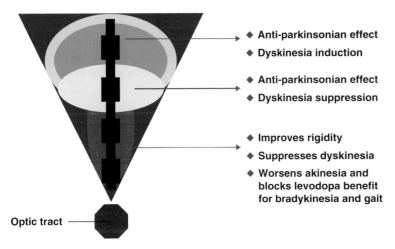

◆ Anti-parkinsonian effect
◆ Dyskinesia induction

◆ Anti-parkinsonian effect
◆ Dyskinesia suppression

◆ Improves rigidity
◆ Suppresses dyskinesia
◆ Worsens akinesia and
  blocks levodopa benefit
  for bradykinesia and gait

Optic tract

Figure 7.3 Dorsal versus ventral globus pallidus internus (GPi) stimulation.

Dorsal stimulation of the globus pallidus produces a marked anti-parkinsonian effect and may induce rather than suppress dyskinesia (similar to STN stimulation); these effects may actually be due to stimulation of the globus pallidus externa (GPe).[20] Ventral simulation may worsen akinesia and block the beneficial effects of levodopa on bradykinesia and gait, while improving rigidity and markedly suppressing dyskinesia. As a result, the middle of the pallidum is probably the optimal site for globus pallidus stimulation, taking advantage of these two divergent effects.

Determination of efficacy on off-period parkinsonism

1. Baseline assessment and testing of monopolar stimulation is similar to thalamic stimulation.

   (a) Test stimulation for each electrode in the monopolar mode at an amplitude slightly below that noted to induce persistent adverse effects. The beneficial effect can be evaluated using a focused motor examination (assessing, for example, contralateral limb rigidity and motor speed) or can be rated more formally using portions of the UPDRS motor scale. Make a note of stimulation-induced dyskinesia, since this may indicate excessive stimulation current spread dorsally. If stimulation-induced dyskinesia is present, rate the improvement in parkinsonism and then slowly reduce the voltage to optimize the amplitude that does not induce dyskinesia before rating the improvement in parkinsonism again.

   (b) Prior to assessing the effects of stimulation with the next electrode, turn stimulation off and perform a quick motor exam to ensure that carry-over effects from stimulating with the previous electrode have largely washed out in order to establish the effects of stimulation at the next electrode on the DBS lead. Unlike in the thalamus, effects of GPi DBS often do not subside immediately after stimulation has been turned off and may not become fully developed immediately after turning stimulation on.

   (c) Repeat the above process using the other DBS lead (for bilaterally treated patients).

2. Decide which one (or two) electrodes provided the best anti-parkinsonian effects with monopolar stimulation. If stimulation-induced adverse effects prevent attainment of adequate parkinsonian motor symptom suppression, then explore bipolar stimulation by testing the best electrode in combination with those adjacent to it using the same methodology as used for monopolar stimulation. If dyskinesia was induced with monopolar stimulation, it may be necessary to use monopolar or bipolar stimulation using more ventrally located electrodes.

3. Rank in order the electrode configurations that provide the best anti-parkinsonian benefit for each side.

73

4. At the end of each programming session, send the patient home on the optimal settings thus far determined.

Determination of efficacy on drug-induced dyskinesia

For GPi DBS, it is important to verify the absence of a levodopa-blocking effect and adequate dyskinesia suppression once the best parameters to improve off-period parkinsonism have been determined. As mentioned above, this is often best performed in the afternoon after at least two doses of medication have been ingested by the patient and they are fully "on."

1. Assess dyskinesia on the optimal settings that improved off-period parkinsonism (as determined above). If dyskinesia is adequately suppressed and there is no worsening of bradykinesia and gait or shortening of the duration of levodopa benefit with stimulation, no further programming is required and the present settings are optimal.

2. If dyskinesia is insufficiently suppressed, determine the best overall electrode configuration for dyskinesia suppression that does not block the beneficial effects of levodopa; this can be accomplished by examining for dyskinesia, bradykinesia, and gait using each of the other two or three electrode configurations that provided reasonably good (though perhaps not optimal) improvement of off-period parkinsonism. Stimulating with more ventrally located electrodes commonly improves dyskinesia suppression. As a result, the best overall final electrode configuration for some patients is a compromise that provides the best combination of improvement in off-period parkinsonism and on-period dyskinesia suppression, without worsening on-period parkinsonism.

Delayed stimulation and medication adjustment

As with thalamic stimulation, optimal stimulation parameters remain fairly stable by one month postoperatively, and only minor adjustments (such as slightly increasing the amplitude) may be necessary beyond three months. Unlike thalamic stimulation in essential tremor, tolerance or habituation has not been observed with GPi DBS in PD. Anti-parkinsonian medication doses and regimen usually do not require significant changes with GPi DBS. In patients with marked levodopa sensitivity and disabling dyskinesia preoperatively, the anti-dyskinetic effects of GPi stimulation may allow higher levodopa doses. Some clinicians do report being able to lower dopaminergic medication doses in patients treated with GPi DBS.

STN DBS programming algorithm (Figure 7.4)

The initial programming methodology is the same as for GPi DBS, except for pulse width, which is usually set to be 60 μs as a starting point; amplitude is set to 0 V and frequency to between 130 and 160 Hz. Stimulation-induced adverse effects expected in the region of the STN are catalogued in Table 7.2.

Determination of efficacy on off-period parkinsonism

1. Baseline assessment and testing of monopolar stimulation follows the same principles as for GPi DBS.

   (a) STN stimulation generally improves rigidity and tremor quickly (in less than one minute). Although the majority of improvement in bradykinesia gradually builds over several minutes, maximal improvement may take several hours. Off-period dystonia is generally improved within minutes of initiating effective stimulation. Dyskinesia may be induced after minutes to days of chronic STN stimulation in the absence of anti-parkinsonian medication. The presence of stimulation-induced dyskinesia is an excellent sign that a well-located electrode has been used for stimulation and suggests that parkinsonism can be maximally improved. If stimulation-induced dyskinesia is present, rate the improvement in parkinsonism and then slowly reduce the voltage to optimize the amplitude that does not induce dyskinesia before rating the improvement in parkinsonism again. The maximal anti-parkinsonian effect of STN stimulation correlates with that achievable by high-dose levodopa therapy, with the exception that tremor may be improved more by

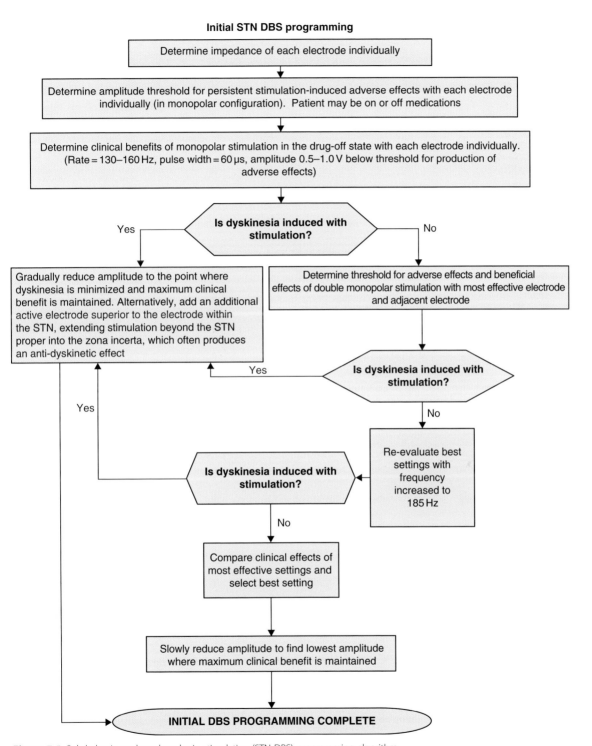

Figure 7.4 Subthalamic nucleus deep brain stimulation (STN DBS) programming algorithm.

75

Table 7.2 Adverse effects of stimulating different anatomical sites in the vicinity of the subthalamic nucleus

Anatomical location	Adverse effect	Habituation	Mechanism/comments	Management
(Numbers for structures correspond to Figure 7.5)				
(1) Corticospinal tract (anterior/lateral to STN)	Tonic muscle contraction	None		Reduce amplitude, change to bipolar electrode configuration, or change stimulating electrode
(1) Corticobulbar tract (lateral to STN, but more medial than corticospinal tract)	Dysarthria	None		Reduce amplitude, change to bipolar electrode configuration, or change stimulating electrode
	Hypophonia		In addition to being caused by spread of stimulation to corticobulbar tract, may be due to excessive levodopa reduction	Examine speech off stimulation after high dose levodopa to determine if worsening of speech is due to drug reduction. Then turn on stimulation to determine if current spread to corticospinal tract is further worsening hypophonia
(2) Medial lemniscus (medial and posterior to STN)	Paresthesia	Seconds		Initially, paresthesia is transient, allowing further escalation in amplitude of stimulation until the point at which persistent paresthesia occurs
(3) Fascicles of oculomotor nerve (inferomedial to STN)	Diplopia	Days to weeks		Reduce amplitude, change to bipolar electrode configuration, or change stimulating electrode (to more superior electrode)
(4) Hypothalamus	Flushing, perspiration	Minutes to hours	Accompanied by feeling of heat	Change electrode or very slowly increase amplitude if the most effective electrode produces this effect to allow for habituation
(5) SNr	Levodopa blocking effect, depression, worsened akinesia	None	May be similar to that seen with ventral GPi stimulation, in which there is improvement in rigidity and dyskinesia but worsening of akinesia	Reduce amplitude, change to bipolar electrode configuration, or change stimulating electrode (to more superior electrode)
(6) Red nucleus	Dysequilibrium and gait ataxia without limb ataxia	None		Reduce amplitude, change to bipolar electrode configuration, or change stimulating electrode. Drug increase often also required
(7) Inferior portion of STN	Limbic (emotional, affective) effects			

Notes: GPi, globus pallidus internus; SNr, substantia nigra reticulate; STN, subthalamic nucleus.

stimulation.[10,23,52] Therefore, the preoperative "best on" level of function can only slightly be improved by the combination of STN stimulation and anti-parkinsonian drug therapy, whereas the preoperative "off" level of function is typically substantially improved.[10,23]

    (b) Prior to assessing the effects of stimulation with the next electrode, turn stimulation off and wait a few seconds to minutes to avoid carry-over effects from stimulation with the previous electrode.

    (c) Repeat the above process using the other side (for bilaterally treated patients).

2. Decide which one (or two) electrodes provide the best anti-parkinsonian effects with monopolar stimulation and begin double monopolar stimulation, and if necessary bipolar stimulation, by testing the best electrode in combination with those adjacent to it using the above methodology.

3. Increase rate to 185 Hz and re-evaluate the best settings thus far determined if no dyskinesia has been induced and the benefit achieved has not been at least equal to that seen with levodopa administration.

4. Rank order the electrode configurations that provided the best anti-parkinsonian benefit for each side.

5. At the end of each programming session, send the patient home on the optimal settings thus far determined. Patients must be warned about the possibility of developing significant delayed-onset dyskinesia and should have a plan for medication reduction and/or reducing or turning off stimulation should this occur.

Identifying the nature of the adverse effects from stimulating the STN region allows one to determine the relative location of each of the electrodes to adjacent structures and appropriate management (Table 7.2 and Figure 7.5). There are a number of adverse effects that can be induced by spread of stimulation outside of the intended target. Adverse effects that rapidly habituate (e.g., paresthesia) do not prevent further increase in stimulation if needed, while adverse effects that do not habituate (e.g., tonic muscle contraction) require a reduction or change in stimulation.

Determination of efficacy on drug-induced dyskinesia

STN stimulation and dopaminergic therapy have an additive effect in inducing dyskinesia, and dyskinesia reduction with STN DBS occurs primarily as a result of drug reduction.[53] Therefore, we generally reduce anti-parkinsonian medication by one-half when beginning chronic STN stimulation, though many clinicians proceed with medication reduction at a slower pace.

Periodic "on-drug" examinations are needed to determine the severity of dyskinesia. Anti-parkinsonian medication is usually reduced as stimulation is increased over days to weeks, depending on the sensitivity of the patient in developing stimulation-induced dyskinesia. Therefore, the presence of significant on-period dyskinesia usually necessitates further drug reduction (or less commonly reduction of stimulation intensity). In contrast, suboptimal effect on parkinsonism without dyskinesia suggests that either anti-parkinsonian medication or stimulation should be increased. If a direct anti-dyskinetic effect of stimulation is noted, one is likely stimulating the substantia nigra reticulata (SNr) below the STN or Zi above the STN.[53]

Indeed, inclusion of an additional active electrode superior to the electrode within the STN, extending stimulation beyond the STN proper into the Zi, often imparts an anti-dyskinetic effect. This can be a highly effective strategy for achieving maximal anti-parkinsonian and anti-dyskinetic effects.

Long-term stimulation, medication, and patient management issues

In the first two to three months postoperatively, the effects of STN stimulation may seem to wane as the micro-lesion effect associated with surgery diminishes. This can be managed by slightly increasing stimulation intensity (accomplished by increasing the amplitude or pulse width or by the addition of another active electrode). If stimulation-induced adverse effects prevent optimal symptom control, then changing stimulation to an adjacent electrode or using a bipolar electrode configuration for

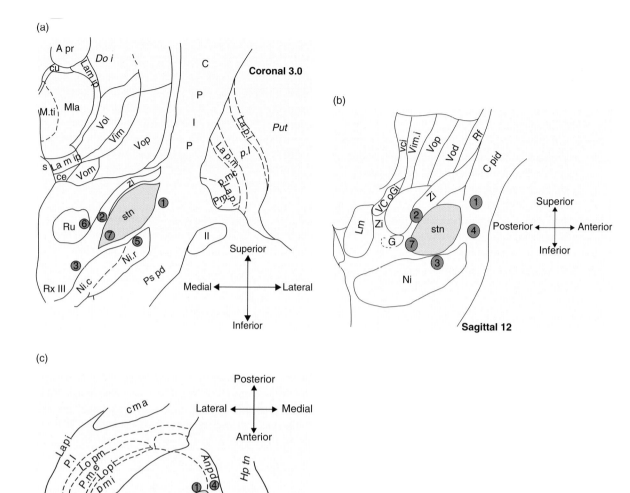

Figure 7.5 Coronal (a), sagittal (b), and axial (c) sections through the subthalamic nucleus region adapted from the Schaltenbrand–Wahren atlas. Refer to Table 7.2 for description of anatomical sites indicated by each number in the figure and the adverse effects of stimulating each location.

stimulation should be considered. If desired improvement is still not achievable, the electrode is likely suboptimally positioned and dopaminergic therapy should be increased. Stimulation settings remain relatively stable in the majority of patients after three months. An average reduction of 50% of

dopaminergic therapy is achieved at 1-year follow up.[3,23,28,54] A small minority of patients are able to discontinue all anti-parkinsonian medication. We prefer to first reduce levodopa, while maintaining continuous dopaminergic stimulation with a long-acting dopamine agonist. Some other clinicians prefer the opposite strategy, since levodopa dosing alone can be quickly and easily changed. With drug reduction and continuous STN stimulation, reduction of dyskinesia gradually increases, allowing a corresponding increase in stimulation. The use of the patient programmer for patients who live a long distance from the DBS center can allow patients to achieve this increase with less travel. Patients with severe preoperative dyskinesia are more apt to develop severe stimulation-induced dyskinesia or even stimulation-induced dystonia. Stimulation-induced dystonia must be differentiated from tonic muscle contraction (by its development over minutes rather than seconds after starting stimulation) and from off-period dystonia. As a result, extremely slow increases in stimulation over weeks may be necessary to allow adaptation to stimulation. In the most extreme cases, the therapeutic window between relief of parkinsonism and induction of disabling dyskinesia or dystonia is too narrow to permit effective stimulation. Use of proximal or distal contacts further from the center of the target and often with bipolar stimulation to reduce current diffusion frequently widens the therapeutic window and thus allows a slow increase in stimulation amplitude in conjunction with chronic drug reduction. Furthermore, as previously noted, in many patients stimulating just above the STN in the Zi may have effects similar to GPi DBS, providing a direct anti-dyskinetic effect.

Reduction in dopaminergic medication may unmask symptoms of restless legs syndrome (RLS) in patients who have previously never complained of such symptoms.[55] More severe cases may be accompanied by dyskinesia during the day, resembling periodic limb movements of sleep. Although an increase in stimulation may improve these symptoms somewhat, as has been previously reported with pallidotomy,[56] in our experience this usually results in inadequate symptom relief and drug therapy is needed.[55] Reintroduction of controlled release levodopa or dopamine agonists may be very helpful but may significantly increase dyskinesia. In such cases, use of gabapentin, benzodiazepines, or opiates can improve RLS symptoms without inducing dyskinesia.

> Overly aggressive reduction in anti-parkinsonian medication should be avoided, since levodopa also improves non-motor symptoms of PD.

A levodopa withdrawal syndrome of abulia, anhedonia, and depression may result.[53,57,58] Reinstitution of low-dose levodopa up to the threshold that produces mild, non-disabling dyskinesia usually quickly improves these symptoms. For persistent symptoms, or when disabling dyskinesia limits levodopa therapy, the use of selective serotonin reuptake inhibitors can be helpful.[53] Depression due to drug withdrawal must be differentiated from acute stimulation-induced depression due to unintentional stimulation of the SNr below the level of the STN.[59] In such cases, depression immediately improves with discontinuation of stimulation, and greater improvement in parkinsonism is achieved stimulating through a more proximal contact.

Postoperative hypomania or mania, including hypersexuality, may occur with STN stimulation that is highly effective for the motor features of parkinsonism and mimics the euphoria-inducing effects of levodopa.[60–62] Rapid reduction in dopaminergic therapy and, if necessary, stimulation amplitude, or moving stimulation to a more dorsal contact will commonly improve this behavior. Similarly, laughing associated with inappropriate affect has been induced by high stimulation settings in which stimulation spreads to the limbic portion of the STN and is accompanied by stimulation-induced dyskinesia.[63]

Preoperative levodopa-refractory postural instability is unlikely to be substantially improved with STN stimulation. As a result of significant improvement in bradykinesia and speed of gait, falls may actually become more frequent postoperatively. Although this may sometimes be improved with physiotherapy, many patients require a walker to prevent falls.

On the other hand, the late development of increased freezing of gait that occurs because of progression of PD, sometimes years after beginning bilateral STN DBS, is common. Reducing stimulation frequency to 60–80 Hz and increasing voltage to just below the threshold for adverse effects so that the total electrical energy delivered remains approximately unchanged, can improve such gait disorders in some cases. However, mild worsening of upper limb bradykinesia may need to be accepted to achieve this benefit.[64]

PPN stimulation

Stimulation of the PPN for treatment of refractory parkinsonian gait and balance disorders may be beneficial, but only a limited number of case series have been reported. The PPN is part of the midbrain locomotor region, communicates with the basal ganglia and cortico-spinal circuits[13], and has bilateral projections to the STN, in addition to connections with the GPi.[12] Animal models demonstrate that the PPN acts in the initiation and maintenance of locomotion.[11,12] In PD, there is a loss of cells in the PPN region.[12] The abnormal firing pattern of the PPN and improvement seen in non-human primate models of PD with lesioning or stimulation have suggested that PPN DBS in humans may selectively target axial symptoms in PD, such as gait impairment and postural stability. Stefani et al.[14] have published the largest case series to date of six PD patients that underwent simultaneous bilateral STN and bilateral PPN stimulation for six months postoperatively. Combined PPN and STN stimulation leads to a greater improvement in UPDRS motor scores on levodopa compared to stimulation of either single target. Gait and postural stability were especially improved when PPN DBS was added to STN DBS. However, combined PPN and STN DBS was not significantly better than STN DBS alone when off medication. The few reported, small case series of unilateral or bilateral PPN DBS alone without STN DBS have reported variable improvement in fall frequency and other axial symptoms, but generally unimpressive results.[15] Further study of PPN DBS is needed before routine clinical application can be recommended.

Continuous mid-frequency stimulation between 20 and 60 Hz induces motor activity but stimulation greater than 100 Hz suppresses muscle tone. Side effects induced by high frequency or high amplitude stimulation include contralateral paresthesia, unilateral eye movements (oscillopsia), and contralateral warm sensations.[14,15] Stimulation parameters are chosen based on the threshold for these side effects and UPDRS scores.[15] For DBS of the PPN, investigators have suggested stimulation parameters of 1.0–4.0 V, 60–90 μs, and a rate of 20–70 Hz.[14,15]

Conclusion

Obtaining optimal results with DBS requires technical knowledge about stimulation, in addition to detailed knowledge of basal ganglia anatomy and the clinical pharmacology and treatment of PD. Understanding and managing the interaction of stimulation and pharmacological therapy is especially important in patients with PD. Acquiring this knowledge provides an important new tool to those who treat PD.

References

1. Ashby P, Rothwell JC. Neurophysiologic aspects of deep brain stimulation. *Neurology* 2000;**55**(Suppl 6):17–20.

2. Benazzouz A, Hallett M. Mechanism of action of deep brain stimulation. *Neurology* 2000;**55**(Suppl 6):13–16.

3. Pollak P. Deep brain stimulation. Presented at the 52nd Annual Meeting of the American Academy of Neurology. San Diego, CA; 2000: May 1.

4. Caparros-Lefebvre D, Ruchoux MM, Blond S, et al. Long-term thalamic stimulation in Parkinson's disease: postmortem anatomoclinical study. *Neurology* 1994;**44**:1856–60.

5. Benabid AL, Chabardes S, Mitrofanis J, Pollak P. Deep brain stimulation of the subthalamic nucleus for the treatment of Parkinson's disease. *Lancet* 2009;**8**:68–81.

6. Ashby P, Kim YJ, Kumar R, et al. Neurophysiological effects of stimulation through electrodes in the human subthalamic nucleus. *Brain* 1999;**122**:1919–31.

7. Hashimoto T, Elder CM, Okun MS, et al. Stimulation of the subthalamic nucleus changes the firing pattern of pallidal neurons. *J Neurosci* 2003;**23**:1916–23.

8. Kopell BH, Rezai AR, Chang JW, et al. Anatomy and physiology of the basal ganglia: implications for deep brain stimulation for Parkinson's disease. *Mov Disord* 2006;**21**(Suppl):S238–46.

9. Vingerhoets FJG, Villemure JG, Temperli P, et al. Subthalamic DBS replaces levodopa in Parkinson's disease: two-year follow-up. *Neurology* 2002;**58**:396–401.

10. Deuschl G, Schade-Brittinger C, Krack P, et al. A randomized trial of deep-brain stimulation for Parkinson's disease. *N Engl J Med* 2006;**355**:896–908.

11. Hamani C, Stone S, Laxton A, Lozano AM. The pedunculopontine nucleus and movement disorders: anatomy and the role for deep brain stimulation. *Parkinsonism Relat Disord* 2007;**13**:S276–80.

12. Pahapill PA, Lozano AM. The pedunculopontine nucleus and Parkinson's disease. *Brain* 2000;**123**:1767–83.

13. Mazzone P, Lozano A, Stanzione P, et al. Implantation of human pedunculopontine nucleus: a safe and clinically relevant target in Parkinson's disease. *NeuroReport* 2005;**16**:1877–81.

14. Stefani A, Lozano AM, Peppe A, et al. Bilateral deep brain stimulation of the pedunculopontine and subthalamic nuclei in severe Parkinson's disease. *Brain* 2007;**130**:1596–1607.

15. Moro E, Hamani C, Poon YY, et al. Unilateral pedunculopontine stimulation improves falls in Parkinson's disease. *Brain* 2010;**133**(Pt 1):215–24.

16. Mitrofanis J. Some certainty for the "zone of uncertainty"? Exploring the function of the zona incerta. *Neuroscience* 2005;**130**:1–15.

17. Plaha P, Ben-Shlomo Y, Patel NK, Gill SS. Stimulation of the caudal zona incerta is superior to stimulation of the subthalamic nucleus in improving contralateral parkinsonism. *Brain* 2006;**129**:1732–47.

18. Saint-Cyr JA, Trépanier LL, Kumar R, et al. Neuropsychological consequences of chronic bilateral stimulation of the subthalamic nucleus in Parkinson's disease. *Brain* 2000;**123**:2091–108.

19. Lang AE, Houeto JL, Krack P, et al. Deep brain stimulation: preoperative issues. *Mov Disord* 2006;**21** (Suppl 14):S171–96.

20. Saint-Cyr JA, Trépanier LL. Neuropsychologic assessment of patients for movement disorder surgery. *Mov Disord* 2000;**15**:771–83.

21. Limousin P, Speelman JD, Gielen F, Janssens M. Multicentre European study of thalamic stimulation in parkinsonian and essential tremor. *J Neurol Neurosurg Psychiatry* 1999;**66**:289–96.

22. Henderson JM, O'Sullivan DJ, Pell M, et al. Lesion of thalamic centromedian-parafascicular complex after chronic deep brain stimulation. *Neurology* 2001;**56**:1576–9.

23. The Deep Brain Stimulation for Parkinson's Disease Study Group. Deep brain stimulation of the subthalamic nucleus or the pars interna of the globus pallidus in Parkinson's disease. *N Engl J Med* 2001;**345**:956–63.

24. Witjas T, Kaphan E, Azulay JP, et al. Effects of subthalamic nucleus (STN) deep brain stimulation (DBS) on non-motor fluctuation (NMF) in Parkinson's disease. *Neurology* 2001;**56**(Suppl 3):274.

25. Arnulf I, Bejjani BP, Garma L, et al. Improvement of sleep architecture in PD with subthalamic nucleus stimulation. *Neurology* 2000;**55**:1732–4.

26. Hjort N, Ostergaard K, Dupont E. Improvement of sleep quality in patients with advanced Parkinson's disease treated with deep brain stimulation of the subthalamic nucleus. *Mov Disord* 2004;**19**:196–9.

27. Krack P, Pollak P, Limousin P, et al. Opposite motor effects of pallidal stimulation in Parkinson's disease. *Ann Neurol* 1998;**43**:180–92.

28. Pahwa R, Wilkinson SB, Overman J, et al. Bilateral subthalamic stimulation in patients with Parkinson disease: long-term follow up. *J Neurosurg* 2003;**99**:71–7.

29. Welter ML, Houeto JL, Tezenas du Montcel S, et al. Clinical predictive factors of subthalamic stimulation in Parkinson's disease. *Brain* 2002;**125**:575–83.

30. Jarraya B, Bonnet AM, Duyckaerts C, et al. Parkinson's disease, subthalamic stimulation, and selection of candidates: a pathological study. *Mov Disord* 2003;**18**:1517–20.

31. Micheli F, Cersosimo MG, Piedimonte F. Camptocormia in a patient with Parkinson disease: beneficial effects of pallidal deep brain stimulation. Case report. *J Neurosurg* 2005;**103**:1081–3.

32. Nandi D, Parkin S, Scott R, et al. Camptocormia treated with bilateral pallidal stimulation: case report. *Neurosurg Focus* 2002;**12**:ECP2.

33. Yamada K, Goto S, Matsuzaki K, et al. Alleviation of camptocormia by bilateral subthalamic nucleus stimulation in a patient with Parkinson's disease. *Parkinsonism Relat Disord* 2006;**12**:372–5.

34. Sako W, Nishio M, Maruo T, et al. Subthalamic nucleus deep brain stimulation for camptocormia associated with Parkinson's disease. *Mov Disord* 2009;**24**:1076–9.

35. Okun MS, Fernandez HH, Wu SS, et al. Cognition and mood in Parkinson's disease in subthalamic nucleus versus globus pallidus interna deep brain stimulation: the COMPARE trial. *Ann Neurol* 2009; **65**(5):586–95.

36. Iansek R, Rosenfeld JV, Huxham FE. Deep brain stimulation of the subthalamic nucleus in Parkinson's disease. *Med J Aust* 2002;**177**:142–6.

37. Fontaine D, Mattei V, Borg M, et al. Effect of subthalamic nucleus stimulation on obsessive-compulsive disorder in a patient with Parkinson disease. Case report. *J Neurosurg* 2004;**100**:1084–6.

38. Mallet L, Mesnage V, Houeto J-L, et al. Compulsions, Parkinson's disease, and stimulation. *Lancet* 2002;**360**:1302–4.

39. Ardouin C, Voon V, Worbe Y, et al. Pathological gambling in Parkinson's disease improves on chronic subthalamic nucleus stimulation. *Mov Disord* 2006;**21**:1941–6.

40. Bandini F, Primavera A, Pizzorno M, et al. Using STN DBS and medication reduction as a strategy to treat pathological gambling in Parkinson's disease. *Parkinsonsim Relat Disord* 2007;**13**:369–71.

41. Krack P, Pollak P, Limousin P, et al. Subthalamic nucleus or internal pallidal stimulation in young onset Parkinson's disease. *Brain* 1998;**121**:451–7.

42. Volkmann J, Allert N, Voges J, et al. Safety and efficacy of pallidal or subthalamic nucleus stimulation in advanced PD. *Neurology* 2001;**56**:548–51.

43. Okun MS, Rodriguez RL, Foote KD, et al. A case-based review of troubleshooting deep brain stimulator issues in movement and

neuropsychiatric disorders. *Parkinsonism Relat Disord* 2008;**14**:532–8.

44. Uitti RJ, Tsuboi Y, Pooley RA, et al. Magnetic resonance imaging and deep brain stimulation. *Neurosurgery* 2002;**51**:1423–31.

45. Anheim M, Batir A, Fraix V, et al. Improvement in Parkinson disease by subthalamic nucleus stimulation based on electrode placement. *Arch Neurol* 2008;**65**:612–16.

46. Shin M, Lefaucheur JP, Penholate MF, et al. Subthalamic nucleus stimulation in Parkinson's disease: postoperative CT-MRI fusion images confirm accuracy of electrode placement using intraoperative multi-unit recording. *Clin Neurophysiol* 2007;**37**:457–66.

47. Larson PS, Richardson RM, Starr PA, et al. Magnetic resonance imaging of implanted deep brain stimulators: experience in a large series. *Stereotact Funct Neurosurg* 2008;**86**:92–100.

48. Rezai AR, Phillips M, Baker KB, et al. Neurostimulation system used for deep brain stimulation (DBS): MR safety issues and implications of failing to follow safety recommendations. *Invest Radiol* 2004;**39**:300–3.

49. Nutt JG, Anderson VC, Peacock JH, Hammerstad JP, Burchiel KJ. DBS and diathermy interaction induces severe CNS damage. *Neurology* 2001;**56**:1384–6.

50. Mogilner AY, Sterio D, Rezai AR, et al. Subthalamic nucleus stimulation in patients with a prior pallidotomy. *J Neurosurg* 2002;**96**:660–5.

51. Bejjani B, Damier P, Arnulf I, et al. Pallidal stimulation for Parkinson's disease. Two targets? *Neurol* 1997;**49**:1564–9.

52. Krack P, Pollak P, Limousin P, Benazzouz A, Benabid AL. Stimulation of subthalamic nucleus alleviates tremor in Parkinson's disease. *Lancet* 1997;**350**(9092):1675.

53. Krack P, Fraix V, Mendes A, Benabid AL, Pollak P. Postoperative management of subthalamic nucleus stimulation for Parkinson's disease. *Mov Disord* 2002;**17**:S188–97.

54. Schupbach WM, Chastan N, Welter ML, et al. Stimulation of the subthalamic nucleus in Parkinson's disease: a 5 year follow up. *J Neurol Neurosurg Psychiatry* 2005;**76**:1640–4.

55. Kedia S, Moro E, Tagliati M, Lang AE, Kumar R. Emergence of restless legs syndrome during subthalamic stimulation for Parkinson disease. *Neurology* 2004;**63**(12):2410–12.

56. Driver-Dunckley E, Evidente VG, Adler CH, et al. Restless legs syndrome in Parkinson's disease patients may improve with subthalamic stimulation. *Mov Disord* 2006;**21**:1287–9.

57. Houeto JL, Mesnage V, Mallet L, et al. Behavioural disorders, Parkinson's disease and subthalamic stimulation. *J Neurol Neurosurg Psychiatry* 2002;**72**:701–7.

58. Berney A, Vingerhoets F, Perrin A, et al. Effect on mood of subthalamic DBS for Parkinson's disease: a consecutive series of 24 patients. *Neurology* 2002;**59**:1427–9.

59. Bejjani BP, Damier P, Arnulf I, et al. Transient acute depression induced by high-frequency deep-brain stimulation. *N Engl J Med* 1999;**340**(19):1476–80.

60. Kulisevsky J, Berthier ML, Gironell A, et al. Mania following deep brain stimulation for Parkinson's disease. *Neurology* 2002;**59**:1421–4.

61. Romito LM, Raja M, Daniele A, et al. Transient mania with hypersexuality after surgery for high frequency stimulation of the subthalamic nucleus in Parkinson's disease. *Mov Disord* 2002;**17**:1371–4.

62. Herzog J, Reiff J, Krack P, et al. Manic episode with psychotic symptoms induced by subthalamic nucleus stimulation in a patient with Parkinson's disease. *Mov Disord* 2003;**18**:1382–4.

63. Krack P, Kumar R, Ardouin C, et al. Mirthful laughter induced by subthalamic nucleus stimulation. *Mov Disord* 2001;**16**:867–75.

64. Moreau C, Defebvre L, Deste'e A, et al. STN-DBS frequency effects on freezing of gait in advanced Parkinson disease. *Neurology* 2008;**71**:80–4.

Managing dystonia patients treated with deep brain stimulation

Ioannis U. Isaias and Michele Tagliati

Introduction

Successful deep brain stimulation (DBS) therapy depends on the proper implementation of a series of interrelated procedures, including appropriate candidate selection, precise lead placement, and proficient device programming. When indicated, medication adjustments and side effect troubleshooting are other important factors to optimize outcome. Competent postoperative management of DBS patients requires a detailed knowledge of the anatomy and physiology of the target area, general expertise in the treatment of movement disorders, and familiarity with the protocols for setting optimal stimulation parameters.[1] In particular, expert programming of the implanted device is essential to optimize DBS therapy. A well-implanted DBS lead in an appropriately selected patient is useless without the application of proper stimulation settings. This is particularly true for dystonia, as clinical results may take weeks or months to manifest.[2]

In this chapter, we will initially review the elements of anatomy that are required in order to understand and control DBS outcomes and side effects in patients with dystonia. In addition, we will review how to select the five essential features for optimal programming in dystonia: optimal electrode selection and configuration, amplitude, pulse width, and rate.

Anatomical target and best lead location

Although thalamic and subthlamic targets have been occasionally used as DBS targets, in particular for secondary dystonias,[3,4] the vast majority of procedures for dystonia target the globus pallidus (GP). Indeed, DBS of the GP has proven to be a safe and effective treatment for disabling primary dystonia[5,6] and some types of secondary dystonia.[7–10]

The GP is a large cellular mass with a triangular shape in its vertical diameter and appears elongated in its horizontal diameter. The anatomy and functional organization of the GP provide important information for the DBS programmer. The GP is divided into two anatomical segments: internal (GPi) and external (GPe). At the base of the GPi is the optic tract, and medial and posterior to the GPi is the internal capsule; both of these structures are relevant for DBS programming.

> The main efferent fibers from the GPi form the pallidothalamic system and include the ventral anterior nucleus of the thalamus and the fasciculus lenticularis, as well as the ansa lenticularis. These two pathways overlap in the posteroventral GPi,[11] making this area a particularly convenient target for modulating GPi output.

Initial programming

Similar to other DBS indications, in the initial programming session in dystonia it is essential for the clinician to assess each of the electrodes on the DBS lead for beneficial and adverse effects and to determine therapeutic settings. Although a "microlesion" effect (transient change in symptoms due to implantation of the DBS lead alone and not to stimulation) is not routinely seen after GPi DBS in dystonia, it is still common practice to wait two to three weeks following DBS lead implantation before performing initial DBS device programming. In contrast to programming DBS for Parkinson's disease, there is generally no need to withhold dystonia medications

---

before programming, and maintaining the patient's usual medications helps to avoid worsening of dystonic symptoms before the beneficial effects of DBS take effect.

As with all DBS programming at the initial programming session, it is useful to measure and record the impedance for each electrode. Baseline impedance testing provides critical information, verifying the integrity of the device electrical system and providing a reference for future troubleshooting. Each electrode should be checked in monopolar (unipolar) mode using a consistent pulse width, rate, and amplitude. Each DBS device has a range of impedances deemed to be normal; an excessively high impedance suggests an open circuit, and an especially low impedance may indicate a short circuit.

> During initial DBS programming in dystonia, it is particularly important to determine the amplitude threshold for stimulation-induced adverse effects (and clinical benefits, when present), since immediate benefit is often not seen and inference of electrode location relies on the types of adverse effects produced and the level of stimulation required to produce them.

A systematic approach should be used to minimize the many variables, and a database should be created in the patient's medical chart for future adjustments and troubleshooting. The effects of stimulating through each electrode of the DBS lead in a monopolar (unipolar) configuration should be assessed with increasing stimulation amplitude until the patient reports a persistent side effect. This procedure is repeated for each of the four electrodes on the DBS lead. When programming bilaterally, the contralateral side should be assessed independently.

Active electrode choice

One of the challenges of the initial programming in patients with dystonia is the virtual absence of immediate clinical response to stimulation. Therefore, the initial choice of the active stimulating electrode is based on some theoretical assumptions and empirical observations. Many clinicians begin empirically with stimulation in the ventral part of the GPi, just above the optic tract, as this region has been shown to have

antidyskinetic effects in PD.[12] In addition, anatomical and physiological studies in primates show that the sensorimotor territory of the GPi is ventral and posterior.[13,14]

As experience with DBS for dystonia increases, patterns of clinical effects correlating with stimulation in different parts of the GPi are being described, providing further empirical support to the notion that the most posterior and ventral area of the GP should be targeted for stimulation. In one study, active electrode locations associated with robust improvement (>70% decrease in dystonia severity scores) were located near the intercommissural plane, at a mean distance from the pallidocapsular border of 3.6 mm.[15] Using a post-hoc analysis of best outcome, another study reported better improvement for the upper limbs with posteroventral stimulation, whereas for lower limbs anterodorsal stimulation provided equivalent efficacy.[16,17] Finally, a prospective multicenter, double-blind, video-controlled study confirmed that ventral pallidal stimulation, primarily of the GPi or medullary lamina or both, is the optimal method for the treatment of dystonia.[18] However, occasional benefits of bilateral acute dorsal pallidal stimulation, primarily of the GPe,[18] suggest that dorsally located electrodes should not be completely ignored, especially when stimulation using ventral electrodes fails to provide benefit. In our first 30 patients successfully treated with pallidal DBS, electrode 0 (most ventral) was used 15% of the time; electrode 1, 38%; electrode 2, 31%; and electrode 3, 16%.[19] Table 8.1 summarizes active electrode locations reported in major published series.

Electrode configuration

> With very few exceptions,[20] most clinicians have used monopolar (unipolar) electrode configurations for successful pallidal DBS in primary dystonia (Table 8.1).

In our experience, over 90% of patients are treated with DBS in monopolar configuration, using multiple adjacent active electrodes in more than half of the cases. In the remaining patients, electrodes are set in a bipolar or tripolar configuration, a choice usually dictated when intolerable motor side effects occur when stimulating in monopolar mode.[19]

Table 8.1 Pallidal deep brain stimulation parameters used in published clinical series

Author (year)	N	Amplitude	Pulse width	Rate	Active electrodes
Bereznai et al. (2002)[40]	6	1.8–3.5 V	120–180 μs	130 Hz	1 (0 and 2)
Krauss et al. (2003)[41]	6	2.2–4.5 V	210 μs	130–145 Hz	1 and 2
Yianni et al. (2003)[20]	25	4.0–7.0 V	150–240 μs	130–180 Hz	Deepest available (bipolar)
Coubes et al. (2004)[30]	31	0.8–1.6 V	450 μs	130 Hz	1 (2)
Krause et al. (2004)[39]	17	Not given	210 μs	130–180 Hz	Electrode above that producing phosphenes
Starr et al. (2004)[42]	23	2.5–3.6 V	210 μs	185 Hz	2
Vidailhet et al. (2005)[24]	22	2.7–4.7 V		100–185 Hz	Not given
Kupsch et al. (2006)[6]	40	3.2±1.1 V	120 μs	130 Hz	Electrode above that producing phosphenes
Isaias et al. (2009)[19]	30	2.5–3.5 V	150–270 μs	60–130 Hz	Mostly 1 and 2

Stimulation parameters

Optimal practices for the three basic DBS electrical parameters (amplitude, pulse width, rate) have not been established. As previously mentioned, there is a good level of "educated guess" involved in the initial choice of stimulation settings, because apart from dystonic tremor, no immediate improvement is usually observed at the time of initial DBS programming. In addition, there is no consensus on how long a delayed response should be awaited before consideration is given to changing electrode configuration or parameters of stimulation.

The early literature documented excellent results using a very long pulse width, high rate, and amplitude just below the adverse effect threshold,[21,22] though other authors have used parameters more consistent with those used for pallidal stimulation in patients with Parkinson's disease.[23,24] However, use of high stimulation rate (>100 Hz) and prolonged pulse width more rapidly depletes the battery of primary cell neurostimulators, leading to frequent neurostimulator replacements (for example, every 18–24 months). For children and young adults treated with DBS, such frequent surgery to replace neurostimulators poses a significant life-long medical burden. Thus, the use of stimulation parameters that extend neurostimulator battery longevity, or the use of rechargeable neurostimulators with greater battery life, are attractive for these patients.

Amplitude

Amplitude controls the volume of tissue that is affected by the stimulation. The largest experience to date pertains to the use of neurostimulators that provide constant voltage stimulation, allowing delivery of stimulation between 0 and 10.5 V.

> In most cases, adverse effect thresholds (mostly caused by stimulation of the internal capsule) dictate the maximum amplitude; for well-located DBS leads in the posteroventral pallidum, therapeutic amplitudes typically range between 1.0 and 3.5 V (Table 8.1).

Lack of stimulation-related adverse effects above 5.0 V should prompt a re-evaluation of lead position. DBS systems delivering a constant *current* of stimulation have become available more recently, and the benefit of delivering stimulation in this mode remains to be determined.

Pulse width

The pulse width specifies the duration of the electrical pulse used to stimulate the target area. The current required to stimulate a neural element decreases as the pulse width increases. This non-linear relation is described by an inverse exponential function.[1] While amplitude controls the volume of stimulated tissue, pulse width can determine which neuronal elements are recruited within that volume.

Initial experience with pallidal DBS for dystonia promoted the idea that long pulse widths are necessary to guarantee optimal clinical outcome, because stimulation had to "suppress" a large number of cell bodies. As theories of DBS mechanisms of action evolve, this practice has been challenged.

> Many clinicians now use much shorter pulse widths (Table 8.1), and one experimental study reported comparable results in patients randomized for a period of 10 hours to short (60–90 μs), medium (120–150 μs), and long (450 μs) pulse widths.[25]

Rate

The rate, which describes the number of electrical pulses delivered per second, in Hertz (Hz), plays a crucial role in the therapeutic effect of DBS. The beneficial effects of relatively high rates of stimulation have been studied systematically for thalamic and subthalamic stimulation in PD patients.[1] The use of higher rates of stimulation was supported also in dystonia by the results of a study showing a superior response of dystonic symptoms to pallidal DBS as stimulation rate was increased from 50 to 250 Hz.[26]

> However, we have recently documented that for treating dystonia, lower rates of stimulation (60–80 Hz) can be as effective as higher frequencies.[19,27,28]

One of the very first reports describing successful treatment of dystonia with GPi DBS described maximal symptomatic relief with stimulation at 50 Hz, though at a very high pulse width.[29] Nevertheless, lower stimulation rates were abandoned when reports of larger patient series demonstrated marked clinical improvement employing 130 Hz or higher rates and wide pulse widths.[6,15,24,30] Importantly, we have found that clinical outcome is not correlated with the total energy delivered, suggesting that positive results in dystonia do not seem to be dependent on the amount of stimulation delivered but on its quality and location.[19]

In the absence of clear guidelines, the choice of optimal parameters of stimulation for treating dystonia is ultimately left to individual experience. Based on our experience, we routinely start stimulation activating electrode 0 or electrode 1 in monopolar configuration. Amplitude is usually set at 2.0–2.5 V, pulse width at 120 μs, and rate at 60 Hz. Figure 8.1 summarizes some of the basic steps of initial DBS programming for dystonia.

Follow-up programming

Similar to initial programming, follow-up visits should use a systematic approach. An initial review of interim changes (including symptom response, medication changes, and adverse events) should be followed by device interrogation and analysis of where the stimulation parameters are within the therapeutic range established during the initial programming visit. Based on this clinical evaluation, a management plan can be formulated to provide stimulation and/or medication adjustments (Figure 8.2).

> Unless particular adverse effects occur, we usually see patients in follow up approximately one month after initial programming, an interval long enough to observe clinical responses that may guide DBS adjustments.

> When clinical response is absent or minimal, stimulation settings can be systematically adjusted by either increasing amplitude (our preferred choice) or pulse width (up to 210 μs). Alternatively, in order to expand the volume of stimulated tissue, we often find it helpful to activate a second or even third electrode in multi-electrode monopolar configuration. Occasionally, in adult patients, we have also seen additional improvement with slight increases of stimulation rates to 70–90 Hz.[31]

Most patients with dystonia are able to substantially decrease their medications, which are usually relatively ineffective, once the beneficial effect of stimulation is established, although this may take weeks or months to occur.[6,24,32] Medication tapering in dystonic patients with DBS is more an art than a science, and there is no consensus in the literature on this point. We normally start tapering medication as soon as we observe some clear sign of clinical improvement, beginning with the drugs that were least effective according to the patient or their parent. We discuss and design slow tapering schedules, in which elimination of each medication takes weeks or

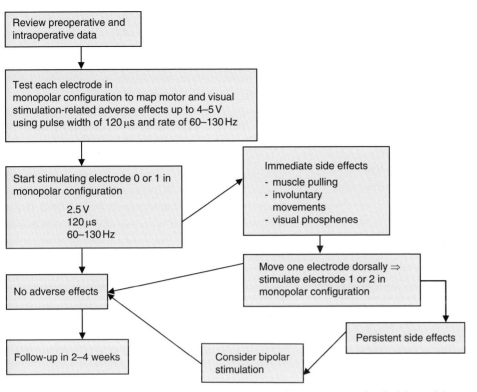

Figure 8.1 Initial deep brain stimulation programming algorithm for dystonia treated with globus pallidus stimulation.

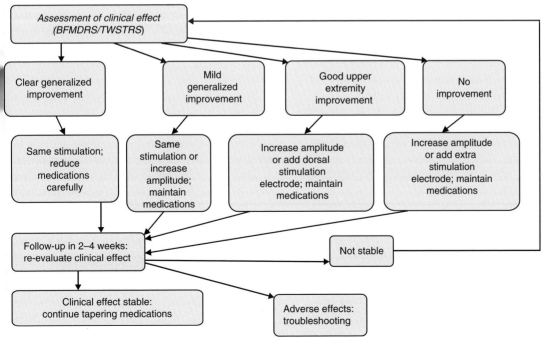

Figure 8.2 Follow-up deep brain stimulation programming algorithm for dystonia treated with globus pallidus stimulation.

months to occur. In our experience, more than half of patients with dystonia are able to discontinue all medications after DBS, while the others are able to reduce their medication requirements by about 60%.[19]

Troubleshooting

Approaches to troubleshooting are discussed in Chapter 9, but issues relevant to patients with dystonia are presented here. There are several reasons for a suboptimal response to DBS therapy, including unresponsive disease, inaccurate lead placement, and suboptimal DBS programming or medication adjustments. Poorly managed expectations can also generate a subjective perception of failure, even when clinical results are objectively apparent. Finally, initial benefit may give way to symptom exacerbations in the presence of technical failures or device malfunctions.

A detailed clinical assessment before and after surgery should be performed to monitor progress.

The widely used Burke–Fahn–Marsden Dystonia Rating Scale (BFMDRS) (Appendix G), the Unified Dystonia Rating Scale (UDRS), and the Dystonia Study Group (DSG) scale showed a similar and acceptable range of internal consistency and inter-rater reliability.[33] The Toronto Western Spasmodic Torticollis Rating Scale (TWSTRS) is available for torticollis (Appendix H).[34] We also recommend videotaping each clinical examination for future reference and comparison with baseline.

On average, the mean improvement of dystonia scores seems to be lower in secondary dystonias in comparison to primary dystonias, with a larger standard deviation, indicating more variable results. Normal MRI is one possible predictor of a favorable outcome for secondary dystonias.[35]

Appropriate DBS lead location is absolutely necessary to achieve optimal results. No amount of expert DBS programming can compensate for a poorly placed lead. Poorly placed DBS leads normally result in unacceptable adverse effects at low levels of stimulation or produce no effect (beneficial or adverse) with test stimulation at high amplitude and pulse width. The nature and localizing value of the adverse effects signaling an inadequate lead location are summarized in Table 8.2. Imaging studies should be obtained in these cases, in order to determine as accurately as possible the location of the DBS lead and for planning revision.

Adequate DBS device programming is crucial for the overall success of DBS. Ideally, patients treated with DBS should receive programming at the same institution, and by the same team that implanted their device. This provides continuity of care and immediate access to information concerning initial programming and lead placement from the operating room. When suboptimal programming parameters are the suspected cause of DBS failure, the history of programming sessions and responses should be reviewed in detail. If this information is not available, a systematic approach, similar to that carried out during initial programming, should be followed (Figures 8.1 and 8.2).

A sudden loss of stimulation efficacy following previous stable symptom control or intermittent side effects suggests a device-related problem. Hardware-related complications generally include lead fracture, extension wire failure, lead migration, skin erosion, foreign body reaction, neurostimulator malfunction, pain, and other less common events.[36] The literature regarding diagnosis, prevention, and treatment of hardware-related DBS complications in dystonia is limited. Hardware-related adverse events, including neurostimulator malfunction, have been reported in long-term follow-up studies. The incidence, ranging from 13 to 40%, seems to be lower in more modern series.[19,37] A high incidence of slipped and fractured DBS leads was reported in patients with cervical dystonia.[38] In a recent review of 30 cases followed for at least 2 years (and up to 8 years), we calculated a 4.9% complication rate per DBS lead–year, which is at the low end of the 4.3–9.5% range reported for other targets and disease populations.[19]

Currently available neurostimulators provide features that may help the programmer in distinguishing device-related problems from other forms of therapeutic failure. These include impedance measurement, battery status indication, and activation and usage counters.

Stimulation-related adverse effects

Table 8.2 describes the most frequent adverse effects related to stimulation of the GPi. Current spread ventrally to the optic tract causes phosphenes (described by patients as bright lights or scintillating visual illusions) and occasionally nausea. Visual side

Table 8.2 Effects caused by globus pallidus region stimulation

Effect	DBS lead is likely	Structure stimulated
Dysarthria at low levels of stimulation	Too posteromedial	Corticobulbar fibers
Tonic muscle contraction at low levels of stimulation	Too posteromedial	Corticospinal fibers
Visual phenomena	Too deep	Optic tract
No effect at high levels of stimulation	Too superior, anterior, or lateral	–

Note: DBS, deep brain stimulation.

effects can be easily avoided by using more dorsal electrodes for stimulation or reducing the amplitude of stimulation.

> The presence of phosphenes may also be helpful in identifying the most ventral part of the GPi; in this case the electrode just above the electrode responsible for producing phosphenes should be used.[6,39]

Electrical current spreading medially or posteriorly into the internal capsule may evoke tonic muscle contraction of contralateral muscles, often associated with dysarthria.[23] Occasionally, involuntary movements (facial or limb dyskinesia) may occur when stimulating the most ventral electrodes in the pallidum. In such cases, amplitude can be reduced or, alternatively, more dorsal electrodes used. If unwanted adverse effects are observed at a low amplitude of stimulation, even lower amplitudes of stimulation combined with increased pulse width can be tested in order to increase current density without further spread of the electrical field. Finally, bipolar or tripolar settings can be used.

References

1. Isaias IU, Tagliati M. Deep brain stimulation programming for movement disorders. In Tarsy D, Vitek J, Starr P, Okun M, eds. *Deep Brain Stimulation in Neurology and Psychiatry*. Totowa, NJ: Humana Press; 2008:361–97.

2. Tagliati M, Shils J, Sun C, Alterman R. Deep brain stimulation for dystonia. *Expert Rev Med Devices* 2004;**1**:33–41.

3. Kleiner-Fisman G, Linliang GS, Moberg PJ, et al. Subthalamic nucleus deep brain stimulation for severe idiopathic dystonia: impact on severity, neuropsychological status, and quality of life. *J Neurosurg* 2007;**107**:29–36.

4. Cersosimo MG, Raina GB, Piedimonte F, et al. Pallidal surgery for the treatment of primary generalized dystonia: long-term follow-up. *Clin Neurol Neurosurg* 2008;**110**:145–50.

5. Vidailhet M, Vercueil L, Houeto JL, et al. Bilateral, pallidal, deep-brain stimulation in primary generalized dystonia: a prospective 3 year follow-up study. *Lancet Neurol* 2007;**6**:223–9.

6. Kupsch A, Benecke R, Muller J, et al. Pallidal deep-brain stimulation in primary generalized or segmental dystonia. *N Engl J Med* 2006;**355**:1978–90.

7. Trottenberg T, Volkmann J, Deuschl G, et al. Treatment of severe tardive dystonia with pallidal deep brain stimulation. *Neurology* 2005;**64**:344–6.

8. Zhang J, Zhang K, Wang Z, Ge M, Ma Y. Deep brain stimulation in the treatment of secondary dystonia. *Chin Med J* 2006;**119**:2069–74.

9. Pretto TE, DAlvi A, Jung Kang U, Penn RD. A prospective blinded evaluation of deep brain stimulation for the treatment of secondary dystonia and primary torticollis syndromes. *J Neurosurg* 2008;**109**:405–9.

10. Sako W, Goto S, Shimazu H, et al., Bilateral deep brain stimulation of the globus pallidus internus in tardive dystonia. *Mov Disord* 2008;**23**:1929–31.

11. Patil AA, Hahn F, Sierra-Rodriguez J, Traverse J, Wang S. Anatomical structures in the Leksell pallidotomy target. *Stereotact Funct Neurosurg* 1998;**70**:32–7.

12. Bejjani BP, Damier P, Arnulf I, et al. Deep brain stimulation in Parkinson's disease: opposite effects of stimulation in the pallidum. *Mov Disord* 1998;**13**:969–70.

13. Iansek R, Porter R. The monkey globus pallidus: neuronal discharge properties in relation to movement. *J Physiol* 1980;**301**:439–55.

14. Parent A, Hazrati LN. Functional anatomy of the basal ganglia. The cortico-basal ganglia-thalamo-cortical loop. *Brain Res Rev* 1995;**20**:91–127.

15. Starr PA, Turner RS, Rau G, et al. Microelectrode-guided implantation of deep brain stimulators into the globus pallidus internus for dystonia: techniques, electrode locations, and outcomes. *J Neurosurg* 2006;**104**:488–501.

16. Tisch S, Zrinzo L, Limousin P, et al. Effect of electrode contact location on clinical efficacy of pallidal deep brain stimulation in primary generalised dystonia. *J Neurol Neurosurg Psychiatry* 2007;**78**:1314–19.

17. Vayssiere N, van der Gaag N, Cif L, et al. Deep brain stimulation for dystonia confirming a somatotopic organization in the globus pallidus internus. *J Neurosurg* 2004;**101**:181–8.

18. Houeto JL, Yelnik J, Bardinet E, et al. French Stimulation du Pallidum Interne dans la Dystonie Study Group. Acute deep-brain stimulation of the internal and external globus pallidus in primary dystonia: functional mapping of the pallidum. *Arch Neurol* 2007;**64**:1281–6.

19. Isaias IU, Alterman R, Tagliati M. Deep brain stimulation for primary dystonia: long-term outcomes. *Arch Neurol* 2009;**66**:465–70.

20. Yianni J, Bain P, Giladi N, et al. Globus pallidus internus deep brain stimulation for dystonic conditions: prospective audit. *Mov Disord* 2003;**18**:436–42.

21. Coubes P, Roubertie A, Vayssiere N, Hemm S, Echenne B. Treatment of DYT1-generalised dystonia by stimulation of the internal globus pallidus. *Lancet* 2000;**355**:2220–1.

22. Cif L, El Fertit H, Vayssiere N, et al. Treatment of dystonic syndromes by chronic electrical stimulation of the internal globus pallidus. *J Neurosurg Sci* 2003;**47**:52–5.

23. Kumar R. Methods for programming and patient management with deep brain stimulation of the globus pallidus for the treatment of advanced Parkinson's disease and dystonia. *Mov Disord* 2002;**17**:198–207.

24. Vidailhet M, Vercueil L, Houeto JL, et al. Bilateral deep-brain stimulation of the globus pallidus in primary generalized dystonia. *N Engl J Med* 2005;**352**:459–67.

25. Vercueil L, Houeto JL, Krystkowiak P, et al. Effects of pulse width variations in pallidal stimulation for primary generalized dystonia. *J Neurol* 2007;**254**:1533–7.

26. Kupsch A, Klaffke S, Kuhn AA, et al. The effects of frequency in pallidal deep brain stimulation for primary dystonia. *J Neurol* 2003;**250**:1201–5.

27. Alterman RL, Miravite J, Weisz D, et al. Sixty hertz pallidal deep brain stimulation for primary torsion dystonia. *Neurology* 2007;**69**:681–8.

28. Alterman RL, Snyde BJ. Deep brain stimulation for torsion dystonia. *Acta Neurochir Suppl* 2007;**97**:191–9.

29. Kumar R, Dagher A, Hutchison WD, Lang AE, Lozano AM. Globus pallidus deep brain stimulation for generalized dystonia: clinical and PET investigation. *Neurology* 1999;**53**:871–4.

30. Coubes P, Cif L, El Fertit H, et al. Electrical stimulation of the globus pallidus internus in patients with primary generalized dystonia: long-term results. *J Neurosurg* 2004;**101**:189–94.

31. Tagliati M, Martin CE, Alterman RL. Optimal pallidal stimulation frequency for dystonia may vary with age. *Mov Disord* 2008;**23**(Suppl 1):S113.

32. Isaias IU, Alterman R, Tagliati M. Outcome predictors of pallidal stimulation in patients with primary dystonia: the role of disease duration. *Brain* 2008;**131**:1895–902.

33. Comella CL, Leurgans S, Wuu J, Stebbins GT, Chmura T. Dystonia Study Group. Rating scales for dystonia: a multicenter assessment. *Mov Disord* 2003;**18**:303–12.

34. Comella CL, Stebbins GT, Goetz CG, et al. Teaching tape for the motor section of the Toronto Western Spasmodic Torticollis Scale. *Mov Disord* 1997;**12**:570–5.

35. Vercueil L, Krack P, Pollak P. Results of deep brain stimulation for dystonia: a critical reappraisal. *Mov Disord* 2002;**17**:89–93.

36. Rezai AR, Kopell BH, Gross RE, et al. Deep brain stimulation for Parkinson's disease: surgical issues. *Mov Disord* 2006;**21**(Suppl 14):S197–218.

37. Blomstedt P, Hariz MI. Hardware-related complications of deep brain stimulation: a ten year experience. *Acta Neurochir* 2005;**147**:1061–4.

38. Yianni J, Nandi D, Shad A, et al. Increased risk of lead fracture and migration in dystonia compared with other movement disorders following deep brain stimulation. *J Clin Neurosci* 2004;**11**:243–5.

39. Krause M, Fogel W, Kloss M, et al. Pallidal stimulation for dystonia. *Neurosurgery* 2004;**55**:1361–70.

40. Bereznai B, Steude U, Seelos K, Botzel K. Chronic high-frequency globus pallidus internus stimulation in different types of dystonia: a clinical, video, and MRI report of six patients presenting with segmental, cervical, and generalized dystonia. *Mov Disord* 2002;**17**:138–44.

41. Krauss JK, Loher TJ, Weigel R, et al. Chronic stimulation of the globus pallidus internus for treatment of non-dYT1 generalized dystonia and choreoathetosis: two-year follow up. *J Neurosurg* 2003;**98**:785–92.

42. Starr PA, Turner RS, Rau G, et al. Microelectrode-guided implantation of deep brain stimulators into the globus pallidus internus for dystonia: techniques, electrode locations, and outcomes. *Neurosurg Focus* 2004;**17**:E4.

Assessing patient outcome and troubleshooting deep brain stimulation

Frandy Susatia, Kelly D. Foote, Herbert Ward, and Michael S. Okun

Introduction

This chapter will review methods of assessing outcomes following deep brain stimulation (DBS) and the approach to troubleshooting problems with DBS that may be responsible for poorer than expected outcomes.

Assessment of DBS outcome

Assessment of clinical outcome following DBS

> Improvement in motor function is the primary outcome assessed in most studies evaluating DBS for movement disorders.

The Movement Disorder Society Unified Parkinson's Disease Rating Scale (MDS-UPDRS) Part III (motor part) is the most extensively reported outcome measure in subthalamic nucleus deep brain stimulation (STN DBS) trials for Parkinson's disease (PD).[1] A trained observer, usually a movement disorder specialist, administers the questionnaire and evaluates the patient according to the 14 items of the scale. Scores range from 0 to 108, with higher scores representing greater impairment.

Prior to surgery, the UPDRS motor subscale is performed in patients in the "off" and "on" medication states. In the medication "off" state, patients abstain from taking PD medications for 12 hours, usually the night prior to the evaluation. In the medication "on" state, patients take PD medication and are assessed in the best "on" state, mostly 30–60 minutes after taking the dopaminergic medications. Since only symptoms responsive to medications are expected to respond to DBS (with the exception of parkinsonian tremor, which may be medication resistant but DBS responsive), improvement of more than 30% is usually required before DBS can be considered.

DBS efficacy can be assessed under different settings, but most effectively in the medication "off" state. The most widely reported evaluation of DBS compares UPDRS scores prior to surgery in the "off" medication state, then at multiple points after surgery in the stimulation "on" and medication "off" state, and then in "on" states (1 – "Off" med/"On" DBS; 2 – "On" med/"On" DBS; 3 – "Off" med/"Off" DBS; 4 – "On" med/"Off" DBS). The outcome is usually reported as the percent improvement over the baseline (preoperative) medication "off" state score.[2]

Other measures that can be used to assess clinical outcome include the impact on the Activities of Daily Living Subscale of the UPDRS (UPDRS-ADL) (Part II); motor fluctuations and dyskinesia using UPDRS Part IV; and other subcomponents of the motor scale, such as scale items evaluating tremor, rigidity, akinesia/bradykinesia, postural instability, and gait. Most published studies evaluate results 6–12 months post-surgery. An average motor score reduction of 20–30% in UPDRS scores is expected when motor function is compared at baseline and after unilateral DBS ("off" medication).[3,4] In bilateral DBS, more than 30% improvement is expected, but Weaver et al.[5] reviewed 31 papers involving STN DBS and 14 papers involving globus pallidus internus deep brain stimulation (GPi DBS). They found that motor function improved by an average of 54.3% and 40% after stimulation of STN and GPi, respectively. Both GPi and STN improved the patients' performance of daily living activities by 40%. STN stimulation

Deep Brain Stimulation Management, ed. William J. Marks, Jr. Published by Cambridge University Press.

significantly reduced medication requirement, but this was not observed in GPi stimulation.

Krack et al.'s[6] study of long-term outcome after STN DBS revealed several significant findings. During assessment in "off" medication/"on" stimulation: (1) UPDRS motor scores improved 66% after 1 year and 54% following 5 years; (2) painful dystonia resolved after 1 year, with the benefit persisting for 5 years; (3) tremor improved by 75%, rigidity improved by 71%, and bradykinesia improved by 49%; (4) gait and postural instability were slightly better than baseline at 5 years but did not change significantly from 1 year following DBS; (5) speech improved at 1 year but returned to baseline level after 5 years.

During assessment in the "on" medication/"on" stimulation condition, STN DBS did not improve UPDRS motor and ADL scores, but the duration and severity of dyskinesia was reduced by 71% and 58%, and this improvement persisted at 5 years; medication dose could be reduced approximately 59% in 1 year's time and did not require further dose escalation after 5 years.

Patients with tremor-predominant PD and essential tremor (ET) have dramatic improvement in their tremor rating scale and ADL score almost immediately following ventral intermediate nucleus of the thalamus deep brain stimulation (Vim DBS) surgery and persisting at long-term follow up ranging from 18–49 months. However, for PD patients, improvements in overall motor scores were not persistent (since stimulation at the Vim target only treats tremor and not other parkinsonian motor features).[7,8]

Assessment of patient quality of life following DBS

Assessment of outcome after DBS includes measurement of: (1) impairment; (2) disability; (3) health-related quality of life (HRQL); and (4) quality of life (QOL). Determination of QOL and HRQL uses patient interviews or questionnaires to reflect patients' global impression of their health or well being.[9] HRQL is thought to be the most useful measure of outcome for DBS.

HRQL is defined as "the capacity to perform the usual daily activities for a person's age and major social role."[10] HRQL reflects functional status rather than disability and assesses if the patient is well enough to be able to perform certain activities. HRQL is less subjective than other measurements of QOL.

The World Health Organization (WHO) defines QOL as an "individual's perceptions of their position in life in the context of the culture and value systems in which they live, and in relation to their goals, expectations, standards, and concerns."[11] QOL determines patient-oriented outcomes. However, it is subject to inconsistencies in patients' understanding of QOL, thereby preventing it from wide use as a measurement of outcome.

Several generic HRQL measurements can be used to determine the effect of medical intervention in PD, such as the Medical Outcome Study Short Form-36 (SF 36),[12–15] Nottingham Health Profile (NHP),[16,17] the Sickness Impact Profile (SIP),[18] and the EuroQol (EQ-5D) (Table 9.1). These compare HRQL among different diseases and between diseased and healthy populations. However, these do not include items highly specific for a disease.

To date, at least six different PD-specific HRQL scales have been developed (Table 9.2), one of which was specifically designed for patients who have undergone DBS.[19] These instruments are more sensitive to small changes in function and improvements due to treatment.

Quality of Life Satisfaction – Deep Brain Stimulation (QLSm-DBS) Scale

The Quality of Life Satisfaction – Deep Brain Stimulation (QLSm-DBS) Scale evaluates the impact of DBS on PD. It was derived by adding two modules to the basic Quality of Life Satisfaction (QLS) Questionnaire. The QLS Questionnaire rates the importance to the patient and his or her satisfaction with various aspects of life. Higher scores represent better HRQL. The first module, Questions on Life Satisfaction – Movement Disorder (QLSm-MD), deals with domains of function affected by movement disorders. The second, QLSm-DBS, covers items regarding the neurostimulator.[20] Both modules take approximately 10–40 minutes to administer.

The first module (QLSm-MD) consists of 12 domains: (1) controllability of movement; (2) absence of dizziness/steadiness when standing and walking; (3) hand dexterity; (4) articulation/speech fluency; (5) ability to swallow; (6) absence of false body sensation; (7) bladder/bowel function; (8) sexual function;

Table 9.1 Generic health-related quality of life (HRQL) measures in Parkinson's disease[16,18,155–163]

Scale	Short Form-36* (SF-36)	Nottingham Health Profile (NHP)	Sickness Impact Profile (SIP)	EuroQol (EQ-5D)
No. of domains and domain names	8 domains: vitality, physical functioning, bodily pain, general health perceptions, physical role functioning, emotional role functioning, social role functioning, mental health	Part I: 6 domains: pain, physical mobility, emotional reactions, energy, social isolation, sleep. Part II contains 7 general yes/no questions concerning daily living problems	12 domains: sleep and rest, eating, work, home management, recreation and pastimes, ambulation, mobility, body care and movement, social interaction, alertness behavior, emotional behavior, communication	5 domains: Pain/discomfort, mobility, usual activity, self care, anxiety/depression
Scoring	Sum the responses in each scale from the SF-36. Each scale is directly transformed into a 0–100 scale on the assumption that each question carries equal weight. Higher scores indicate better HRQL	Parts I and II: each question is assigned a weighted value, which gives a range of possible scores from 0 (no problems at all) to 100 (presence of all problems within a dimension). Lower scores represent better HRQL	Lower scores represent better HRQL. The general adult population has an SIP score of about 5, whereas an SIP score of 20 indicates the need for substantial daily care, and a score of greater than 30 indicates the need for almost complete care	Lower scores represent better HRQL. Higher scores on the VAS represent better imaginable health
Mode of administration	Self-administration	Self-administration	Self-administration	Self-administration
No. of items	36	38	136	5
Completion time (approx.)	5–10 minutes	5–10 minutes	20–30 minutes	5 minutes
Internal consistency reliability	0.80–0.95	0.83–0.90 except for sleep, energy, and social isolation	NA	NA
Test–retest reliability	NA	0.85	NA	NA

Notes: Medical Outcomes Study Short Form-36.
Several aspects of psychometrics have not yet been investigated in the field of Parkinson's disease and are marked NA (not available).

(9) sleep; (10) mentation (memory); (11) functional independence; and (12) inconspicuousness of illness. The second module (QLSm-DBS) consists of 5 domains: (1) reliability of the stimulator; (2) inconspicuousness of the stimulator; (3) independent handling of the stimulator; (4) physician care (quality and availability); and (5) absence of bodily symptoms/side effects of the neurostimulation. QLSm-MD and QLSm-DBS have good reliability and validity.[20]

Quality of Life in Essential Tremor Questionnaire (QUEST)

The Quality of Life in Essential Tremor Questionnaire (QUEST) is a newly developed ET-specific QOL measurement with good reliability. It has 30 items, consisting of 5 domains: (1) physical; (2) psychosocial; (3) communication; (4) hobbies/leisure; and (5) work/finance. It is a quick, self-administered questionnaire that can be completed in approximately 5–10 minutes. Higher scores correspond to more impairment.[21]

Table 9.2 Disease-specific health-related quality of life (HRQL) measures for Parkinson's disease[19,20,163–169]

Scale	PDQ-39	PDQL	PDQUALIF	PIMS	QLSm-MD	QLSm-DBS
No. of domains and domain names	8 domains: mobility, activity of daily living, emotional well-being, stigma, social support, cognition, communication, and bodily discomfort	4 domains: parkinsonian symptoms, systemic symptoms, social function, and emotional function	7 domains: social/role function, self-image/sexuality, sleep, outlook, physical function, independence, and urinary function	10 domains: self-positive, self-negative, family relationships, community relationships, safety, leisure, travel, work, financial security, and sexual activity	12 domains for movement disorders: controllability of movement, absence of dizziness/steadiness when standing and walking, hand dexterity, articulation/speech fluency, ability to swallow, absence of false body sensation, bladder/bowel function, sexual function, sleep, mentation (memory), functional independence, and inconspicuousness of illness	5 domains for DBS: reliability of the stimulator, inconspicuousness of the stimulator, independent handling of the stimulator, physician care (quality and availability), and absence of bodily symptoms/side effects of the neurostimulation
Scoring	Lower scores represent better HRQL	Higher scores represent better HRQL	Lower scores represent better HRQL	Lower scores represent better HRQL	Higher scores represent better HRQL	Higher scores represent better HRQL
Mode of administration	Self-administration	Self-administration	Self-administration	Self-administration	Self-administration	Self-administration
No. of items	39	37	33	10	29	17
Completion time	20–30 min	15–20 min	10–15 min	10–20 min	10–40 min	10–40 min
Internal consistency reliability	Total scale: 0.84–0.94 Subscales: 0.72 (bodily discomfort) to 0.95 (mobility)	Total scale: 0.94 Subscales: 0.80 (systemic symptoms) to 0.87 (emotional functioning)	Total scale: 0.89 Subscales: 0.55 (physical function) to 0.85 (social function)	Total scale: 0.90	Total scale: 0.87	Total scale: 0.73
Test-retest reliability	Good, except for social support	NA	0.88 (overall)	0.72	NA	NA

Notes: DBS, deep brain stimulation; PDQ-39, Parkinson's Disease Questionnaire; PDQL, Parkinson's Disease Quality of Life Questionnaire; PDQUALIF, Parkinson's Disease Quality of Life Scale; PIMS, Parkinson's Impact Scale; QLSm-MD, Quality of Life Questions on MD; QLSm-DBS, Quality of Life Questions on Satisfaction - Movement Disorder.

Quality of life for dystonia

There is no established disease-specific quality of life measure for dystonia as of yet. Most of the QOL published papers use generic QOL questionnaires.[22–26]

Assessment of neuropsychiatric and neuropsychological outcome following DBS

Neurobehavioral changes following STN DBS and GPi DBS have been increasingly reported.[27–29] Neuropsychiatric problems have been more frequently reported after STN DBS, but they may occur in all targets.[27] A neuropsychological and neuropsychiatric examination should be performed in DBS candidates to identify problems and predisposing factors. All active psychiatric problems should be treated prior to surgical intervention,[28,30,31] because these may worsen following DBS surgery and impede best outcomes.

Several neuropsychiatric and neuropsychological batteries can be used to measure outcome after DBS surgery and are listed in Table 9.3. Declines

Table 9.3 Neuropsychological and neuropsychiatric screening tests commonly utilized for assessment of deep brain stimulation surgery outcome.

Global cognition	Folstein Mini Mental Status Examination (MMSE),[170] Mattis Dementia Rating Scale,[171] Weschler Abbreviated Scale of Intellegence (WASI)[172]
Executive cognitive functions	
Behavioral control	Prehension behavior[173]
Conceptualization	Similiarities/Wechsler Adult Intelligence Scale (WAIS-III),[172] Wisconsin Card Sort Test (WCST)[174]
Processing speed	Trail Making Test B (TMT-B),[175,176] Animal Fluency[177]
Set activation	Verbal Fluency (C, F, L)[178]
Set shifting	Trail Making Test B (TMT-B)[175,179,180]
Set maintenance	Stroop Test,[181,182] Odd Man Out Test[183]
Working memory	Digit Span Test,[184] Spatial Span (CANTAB),[185] Digit Ordering Test,[186] Paced Auditory Serial Addition Test (PASAT)[187,188]
Memory	Weschler Memory Scale-III (WMS-III),[184] Hopkins Verbal Learning Test (HVLT),[189,190] Rey Auditory and Verbal Learning Test (RAVLT),[191,192] Free and Cued Recall Test[193]
Problem solving	Tower of London Test,[194] Delis–Kaplan Executive Function System (D-KEFS)[195,196]
Instrumental cognitive functions	
Language	Boston Naming Test (BNT),[197,198,199] Letter and Category Fluency[200]
Visuo-constructive	Clock Drawing Test (CDT)[201]
Visuo-spatial	Judgement of Line Orientation Test (JLOT), Benton Line Orientation Test (BOT),[202] Cube Analysis (Visual Object and Space Perception Battery/VOSP),[203] Hooper Visual Organization Test[204,205]
Visuo-perceptive	Benton Facial Recognition Test,[206] Fragmented Letters (Visual Object and Space Perception Battery/VOSP)[203]
Neuropsychiatric functions	
Apathy	Apathy Evaluation Scale (AES),[207] Lille Apathy Rating Scale (LARS)[208]
Anxiety	Hamilton Anxiety Scale (HAM-A)[209]
Depression	Montgomery–Asberg Depression Rating Scale (MADRS),[210] Hamilton Depression Rating Scale (HAM-D),[210,211] Beck Depression Inventory (BDI),[212] Geriatric Depression Scale (GDS-15),[213] Zung Self Rating Depression Scale (ZSRDS)[214,215]
Mania	Mania Rating Scale (MRS)[216]
Mood	Visual Analog Mood Scale (VAMS)[217]
Obsessive Compulsive	Yale–Brown Obsessive Compulsive Scale (Y-BOCS)[218–220]
Psychotic symptoms	Neuropsychiatric Inventory (NPI),[221] Parkinson Psychosis Questionnaire (PPQ6)[222]

in global cognitive function,[32–34] executive function,[34–36] memory and learning,[37–39] and verbal fluency,[29,40] including semantic, phonemic, and syllabic issues, can present as early as three months following STN DBS.[32,34,39,41,42]

Approach to DBS troubleshooting

There are several reasons why patients may not experience expected levels of improvement following DBS surgery, including surgery-related complications (e.g., intracerebral hemorrhage, deep cerebral venous hemorrhage infarction, seizure, sterile seroma, pulmonary embolism, pneumonia, perioperative confusion, suboptimal lead placement), device-related issues (e.g., infection, skin erosion, electrode or wire break, lead migration, neurostimulator migration, neurostimulator malfunction, pain in neurostimulator region), and stimulation-related issues (e.g., paresthesias, muscle contraction, postural instability, dyskinesia, dysarthria, abnormal eye movement, apraxia of eyelid opening, hypomania, depression, psychosis, anxiety, sialorrhea, visual phenomena). Other possible reasons for a lack of improvement after DBS surgery include disease progression, being a poor DBS candidate, lack of a multidisciplinary team to appropriately manage the patient, unrealistic patient expectations or failure to achieve patient expectations, poor access to device programming, improper programming and medication adjustment, tolerance to DBS stimulation, and neuropsychiatric complications.

An important concept in the evaluation and assessment of DBS patients is to utilize a multidisciplinary, or team, approach. This team consists of a movement disorder-trained neurologist and neurosurgeon, physician assistant/nurse DBS programmers, psychiatrists, neuropsychologists, occupational therapists, nutritionists, speech pathologists, social workers, financial counselors, and home care case managers.[31,43]

A patient who has had problems or loss of benefit from DBS implantation should be evaluated carefully (Figure 9.1). This may take several hours or potentially several days. For example, troubleshooting at our center requires a minimum of two days. The first day encompasses a thorough clinical evaluation of the patient, followed by a neuroimaging examination (an MRI scan, if possible). If an MRI is not possible because of an abdominally placed neurostimulator or other reason, a CT scan is performed. The clinical evaluation includes gathering of the patient's personal data, co-morbidities, and implantation data from inside or outside the institution (target, track location, equipment used, whether microelectrode date were acquired, whether there were placement issues in the operating room, whether a proper medication trial was performed, whether neuropsychological evaluations were performed, the DBS parameter settings, specific problems and their timeline in relation to the DBS implant(s), and medication trials and changes). This is followed by a routine physical examination. After that, the patient undergoes either a brain MRI scan (following the DBS device manufacturer's safety guidelines) or a head CT scan. The patient will be asked to discontinue medications at least 12 hours prior to the visit the next day. The DBS leads on the image are measured in three-dimensional space to localize the tip and each electrode of the DBS lead.

On the second day, the patient will have been "off" medication overnight (if a patient with PD) and stimulation will be "on." The patient will first have stimulation-related amplitude thresholds at each electrode on the DBS lead checked for side effects and benefits. Based on this information, DBS reprogramming is then attempted. Patients can be evaluated using the UPDRS if they have PD, the Fahn–Tolosa–Martin Tremor Rating Scale (TRS) if they have tremor, or the Burke–Fahn–Marsden Rating Scale (BFMRS) if they have dystonia. If the DBS lead is mal-located and a revision of the DBS lead is being considered, the patient is referred for a full multidisciplinary evaluation to assess if the revision surgery is appropriate. These team members independently evaluate co-morbidities, risks, and appropriate targets, and then meet to decide on the best management strategy (medications/programming versus lead replacement).

Potential problems/issues and solutions encountered with DBS

Troubleshooting surgery-related complications (Table 9.4)

Assessment and management of surgery-related issues and complications can be challenging in the acute time following DBS implantation surgery,

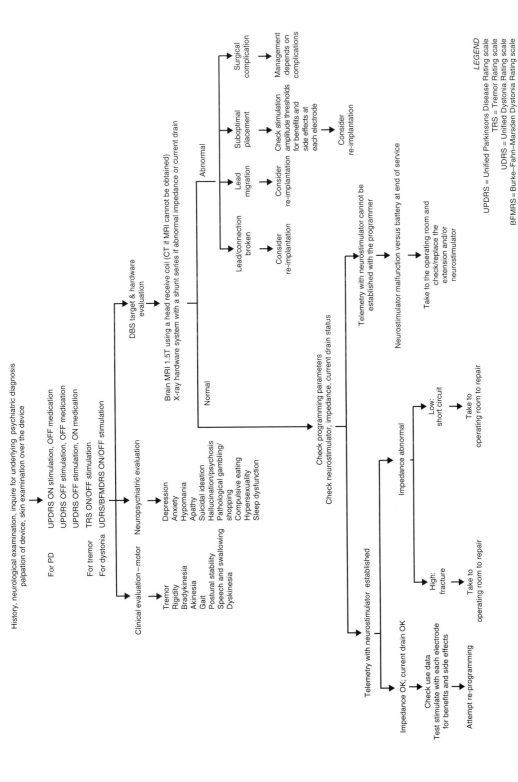

Figure 9.1 Algorithm for assessment and troubleshooting post-deep brain stimulation.

Table 9.4 Frequency of deep brain stimulation complications

DBS complications		Frequency
Surgery-related issues	Intracerebral hemorrhage	1–5%[45,46–49]
	Deep cerebral venous hemorrhage/infarction (delayed)	0.9–2.3%[45,52,223]
	Seizure	3.1%[62]
	Sterile seroma	–
	Pulmonary embolism	0.4–4.9%[63]
	Pneumonia	0.6%[67]
	Perioperative confusion	1–36%[6,69,70]
	Suboptimal lead placement	3.8–12%[45,73]
Device-related issues	Infection	3–10%[48,52,62]
	Skin erosion	2.5–6.45%[48,79]
	Electrode or wire fracture	5.1–18%[48,72]
	Lead migration	5.1%[82]
	Neurostimulator malfunction	18%[72]
	Neurostimulator migration	18%[72]
	Pain in region of neurostimulator	11–36%[80]
Stimulation-related issues	**Vim**	
	Paresthesias	10%[93]
	Muscle contractions	–
	Dysarthria	5–25%[98–100]
	Postural instability/ataxia	3–7%[95,98,100,102,103]
	STN	
	Dyskinesia/hemiballismus	–
	Paresthesias	–
	Muscle contractions	–
	Dysarthria/dysphonia	4–17%[6,105–107]
	Gait/postural instability	–
	Abnormal eye movements/diplopia	–
	Apraxia of eyelid opening	5%[62]
	Neuropsychiatric:	
	Postoperative confusion	1–36%[6,69,70,120]
	Hypomania	4–15%[70,121]
	Anxiety/emotional reactivity	75%[118]
	Suicide attempt/suicide	0.5–2.9%[6,119,124]
	Depression	2.9%[6,119,124]
	Psychosis	11–16%[35]
	Cardiovascular reflexes	48%[129]
	Sialorrhea	–
	Dysphagia	4–8%[107,122,133]
	Hypersexuality	2.4%[134]
	Weight gain	6–100%[6,107,135]
	GPi	
	Muscle contractions	–
	Dysarthria	Rare[70,145]
	Visual phenomena	–

Table 9.4 (cont.)

DBS complications

		Frequency
Other issues	Disease progression	–
	Poor DBS candidate	–
	Lack of the multidisciplinary team to manage patient	–
		–
	Unrealistic patient expectation/failure to achieve patient expectations	–
		–
	Poor access to DBS programming	
	Improper device programming and/or medication adjustment	
	Tolerance	

Notes: DBS, deep brain stimulation; GPi, globus pallidus internus; STN, subthalamic nucleus; Vim, ventral intermedius. DBS complications that have not yet been investigated or reported with clear frequency ranges are marked "–"

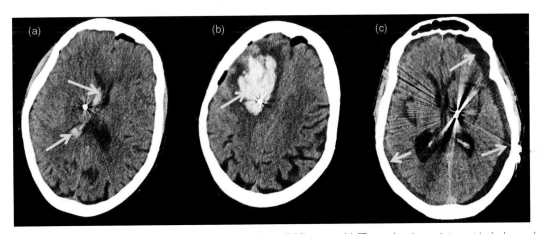

Figure 9.2 Intracranial hemorrhage after deep brain stimulation (DBS) surgery. (a) CT scan showing an intraventricular hemorrhage following DBS lead implant into the right subthalamic nucleus. (b) CT scan showing a large right frontal hemorrhage along the electrode tract following DBS lead implant into the subthalamic nucleus (STN). (c) CT scan showing a left STN DBS lead with bilateral panhemispheric subdural effusions, status post-bilateral posterior craniotomies and evacuation of extra-axial fluid.

mainly since the DBS system often has not been turned on until several weeks after surgery.[44]

Intracerebral hemorrhage/subdural hematoma

Intracerebral hemorrhage (ICH) occurs in approximately 1–5% of DBS cases (Figure 9.2).[45–48] The incidence of ICH seems to be higher in DBS cases performed with microelectrode recording (MER) with multiple electrode passes[49,50] and hypertensive patients, although controversy exists regarding this topic.[51] Bleeding may happen several hours or days after surgery. The risk of bleeding is 3.3% per lead implantation,[52,53] and around 0.6% of patients will suffer permanent neurological deficits.[53,54]

Prevention

Hemorrhagic complications can be prevented by: (1) planning the most appropriate point of entry into the cranium and avoiding puncturing superficial

99

veins and sulci near the entry point; (2) controlling blood pressure pre-, intra-, and postoperatively; (3) screening for coagulopathies or recent use of anti-platelet agents before surgery; (4) giving special precaution to MER use in hypertensive patients who require multiple electrode passes[51]; (5) avoiding performing the procedure on patients who have a respiratory condition that would lead to a severe cough or sneeze in an effort to avoid a sudden increase in intracranial pressure and injury during surgery.[53]

Troubleshooting

Optimize medical management (i.e., maintain airway and ventilation, blood pressure, and intracranial pressure) and neurosurgical preventative interventions. If there is blood noted on the cannula or if deterioration in the level of consciousness occurs and a focal neurological deficit appears, the DBS surgery should be interrupted, and a head CT scan should be performed. If a small bleed is found on the CT scan, this can be managed by leaving the stereotactic frame in place to aid aspiration of the blood. If the bleed is large, a decompressive craniectomy may be needed to prevent brainstem compression and further complications.[55]

Delayed deep cerebral venous bleeding/infarction

Cerebral venous thrombosis (CVT) or hemorrhage may occur when a thrombus forms in the large draining veins that enter the dura mater at the site of a burr hole or when a vein is injured during the DBS procedure. Symptoms include severe headache, seizures, change in mental status, and focal neurological deficit. The severity depends on how severely the thrombus occluded the venous territory, causing venous congestion, and compensation from collateral vessels.[56] Brain MRI venography will show the location of the thrombus in the vein and dural sinus system.[57]

Prevention

CVT can be prevented by detailed surgical planning with a gadolinium brain MRI and the placement of burr holes anterior to the coronal suture to minimize venous infarction. Blood screening for certain risk factors such as hypercoagulable states associated with polycythemia vera, antiphospholipid syndrome, protein S and C deficiencies, antithrombin III deficiency, lupus anticoagulant, Factor V Leiden, sickle cell,

malignancies, etc. prior to surgery may also be helpful in preventing CVT.

Troubleshooting

CVT can be treated by administering an anticoagulant (unfractionated heparin or low molecular weight heparin) to prevent thrombus spread and increase the possibility of recanalization, although whether this should be done is best decided together with a hematologist. Patients should be maintained at an international normalized ratio (INR) of 2.0–3.5 for at least 3 months. Patients with severe risk factors, such as thrombophilia or antiphospholipid syndrome, may require treatment for a longer time. Anti-thrombotic agents and thrombolytics can also be given to manage CVT. Repeated lumbar puncture or the construction of a lumboperitoneal shunt to reduce intracranial hypertension can be performed to treat headache and papilledema.[58] In the rare patient who develops brain herniation and coma, an emergency decompressive hemicraniectomy should be done.[59,60] Antiepileptic drugs should be administered in CVT patients with seizure.[61]

Seizure

The incidence of postoperative seizures after DBS surgery is approximately 3.1%.[62] There are currently no data correlating the number of trajectories inserted with seizure incidence.

Troubleshooting

When a seizure occurs postoperatively, antiepileptic medications should be administered, usually until three to six months postoperatively. The long-term seizure risk is very low.[46,47] It is not recommended to give prophylactic anti-convulsants prior to DBS surgery because they may increase medication-related complications and drug–drug interactions, especially in the elderly population.

Sterile seroma

A seroma is a sterile accumulation of serum in a circumscribed location within the tissue. It is caused by an injury during the surgical procedure that does not fully subside. The remaining serous fluids cause seroma that the body usually absorbs gradually.

Troubleshooting

If the fluid collection does not resolve spontaneously over days or weeks, then drainage by needle puncture may be necessary. If there is any suspicion of an infection, the fluid should be sent for culture analysis.

Pulmonary embolism

Pulmonary embolism (PE) occurs at an incidence of 0.4–4.9% after DBS surgery. The mortality rate ranges from 8.6% to as high as 59.4%.[63] The risk of PE is increased in PD patients because of their immobility. PE should be suspected in patients who experience sudden onset of dyspnea, tachypnea, pleuritic chest pain, cough, and hempotysis.

Prevention

Pneumatic leg compressors should be used in patients with indicators of high risk (for example, heart disease, obesity, polycystemia, paralysis of lower extremities, and forced immobilization). Low molecular weight heparin can also be administered to prevent deep vein thrombosis (DVT) and subsequent PE,[64] in selected cases.

Troubleshooting

Low molecular weight heparin should be administered initially and then shifted to warfarin to achieve an INR between 2.0 and 3.0. If another episode of PE occurs while under warfarin treatment, the INR window may be increased to approximately 2.5–3.5.[65,66]

Pneumonia

Postoperative pneumonia is especially common in PD patients with pre-existing swallowing difficulties that predispose them to aspiration. The incidence rate is approximately 0.6% in the 30 days following DBS surgery.[67]

Troubleshooting

When pneumonia is suspected, appropriate antibiotics should be administered. Piperacillin/tazobactam or imipenem/cilastatin plus vancomycin are appropriate for many moderate to severe pneumonia cases.[68] A culture identifying the organism will give a better rationale for treatment and determine the choice of antibiotics. Often an infectious disease consult is appropriate.

Perioperative confusion

Perioperative confusion is common following STN DBS surgery. The incidence is approximately 1–36%.[6,69,70] Many factors contribute to confusion, including penetration of the frontal lobe, the long duration of surgery, withdrawal of dopaminergic medications, and pre-existing cognitive deficits. Perioperative confusion is usually transient.

Troubleshooting

If confusion is persistent, a full neurological examination and neuroimaging studies should be performed. Additionally, blood studies, urinalysis, preoperative neuroimaging, and baseline neuropsychological testing should be reviewed to search for pre-existing potential risk factors.

Suboptimal lead placement (Figure 9.3)

Suboptimal lead placement is one of the most common causes of DBS failure.[71] Factors that may result in a misplaced lead include poor surgical technique, head movement or frame shift, misinterpretation of MER data, and brain shift.[45,72] The incidence

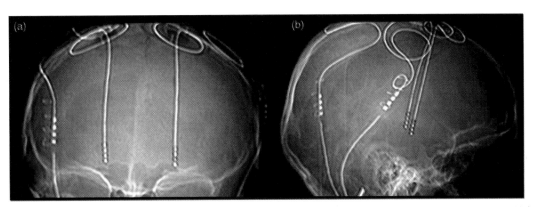

Figure 9.3 Suboptimal deep brain stimulation (DBS) lead location. Plain X-ray, AP (a) and lateral (b), showing suboptimal left DBS lead placement following subthalamic nucleus (STN) DBS surgery. The best imaging technique to identify lead location is MRI, if available.

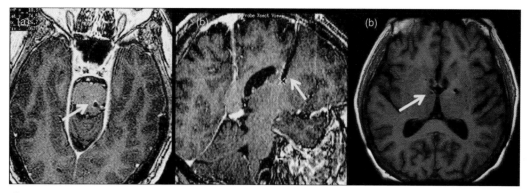

Figure 9.4 Misplaced deep brain stimulation (DBS) lead. (a) Brain MRI in the axial plane showing that the left DBS lead position is too deep beneath the pontomedullary junction. (b) Brain MRI in the sagittal plane demonstrating that the right DBS lead position is too shallow within the periventricular white matter of the centrum semiovale following subthalamic nucleus (STN) DBS surgery. (c) Brain MRI in the axial plane revealing that the right DBS lead is placed too far medial after globus pallidus internus (GPi) DBS surgery.

varies from 3.8 to 12% of patients and from 2.2 to 9% of all procedures.[45,72,73]

Prevention

Suboptimal lead placement can be prevented by: (1) improving surgical technique; (2) confirming DBS lead position during surgery by intraoperative fluoroscopy before and after the lead has been locked by a securing device, and by obtaining a head CT scan/brain MRI postoperatively to confirm the position of the lead[44]; (3) minimizing traction on the brain while fixing the lead.

Troubleshooting

1. Test stimulation amplitude thresholds that produce benefits and side effects for each electrode on the DBS lead and try programming at one month after surgery.
2. Evaluate the lead location using MRI (Figure 9.4), following the safety guidelines of the device manufacturer (a CT scan can be done if there are contraindications to an MRI) and determine the anatomical three-dimensional position of each electrode on the DBS lead.
3. Gather and review all data (clinical assessment, side effects, benefits, lead position) and decide whether there is an electrode that can be used to deliver stimulation and provide benefit.

If the benefit of programming cannot be sustained for more than hours or a few days, or if side effects occur at low stimulation thresholds, a suboptimally located lead should be suspected and replacement of the intracranial lead considered.[44]

Management of device-related issues

Infection (Figure 9.5)

Infection is the most common device-related surgical complication. The incidence ranges from 3 to 10% in most series.[52,62,48,74] In cases of high infection rates (12–15.1%),[48,75] the hospital infectious disease committee should be called in to investigate possible sources within the hospital and its employees. In general, infected DBS systems that involve the brain portion of the lead system need to be removed. Treatment with antibiotics without device removal is not likely to be effective. Leaving an infected lead in place can potentially result in a severe intracranial infection, such as a subdural empyema or brain abscess.

Prevention

Several recommendations have been made for reducing the postoperative infection rate. These include: (1) using strict aseptic surgical methods (e.g., washing the surgical skin site with chlorhexidine)[76]; (2) improving surgical technique (e.g., a curvilinear incision is preferable to evade crossing of the lead anchoring device); (3) reducing surgical time; and (4) using antibiotics (cefazolin).[72,74] The first dose of cefazolin should be given before surgery; the second and third doses after surgery. If the patient is sensitive to cefazolin sodium, one dose of vancomycin

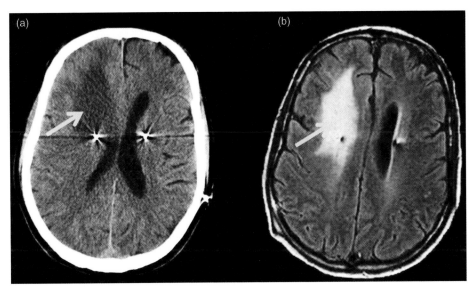

Figure 9.5 Deep brain stimulation (DBS)-related infection. (a) CT scan in the axial plane showing bilateral subthalamic nucleus (STN) DBS implantation and hypodensity in right frontal area (vasogenic edema), which creates right-to-left subfalcine shift. (b) MRI scan in the axial plane showing fronto-parietal edema due to infectious process.

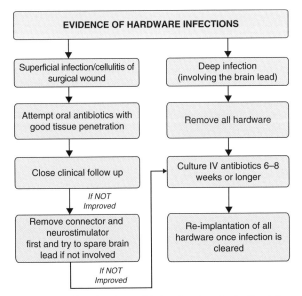

Figure 9.6 Algorithm for troubleshooting deep brain stimulation infections.

hydrochloride can be administered before surgery.[72] The role of shaving off hair to prevent infection is still controversial,[77] and many centers such as ours perform hair-sparing operations with a low infection rate. In case hair needs to be shaved, an electric clipper is preferable to a razor to lower the infection rate.[78]

Troubleshooting (Figure 9.6)

If the infection is superficial and mainly a localized skin infection of the surgical wound, it may be treated with intravenous or even oral antibiotics with adequate tissue penetration. A close clinical follow-up visit must be performed to evaluate the infection. If the infection does not improve with the antibiotics, the extension and neurostimulator should be removed. Repeat the culture and administer the appropriate antibiotics based on the findings of that culture (the antibiotic course should be for six to eight weeks). Implantation of new hardware can be performed once the infection has cleared.

If the infection is deep and involves purulence around the brain lead, it must be treated by immediate removal of the hardware. Perform culture studies and administer a sufficient course of antibiotics (usually at least six to eight weeks) prior to replacement of hardware. In severe cases of deep, purulent infection around the brain lead, it is often prudent to consult an infectious disease specialist.

Skin erosion

Skin erosion occurs mostly at the connector site that joins the DBS lead to the extension. It is usually a late-occurring complication, with an incidence of 2.5–6.5%.[48,79] The original connector used in the past was bulkier, which may have contributed to this

103

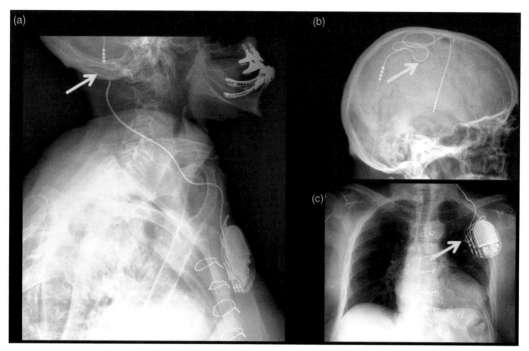

Figure 9.7 Example of a deep brain stimulation (DBS) lead fracture. Plain X-ray film series through the skull, neck, and chest of a "twiddler" patient demonstrating a DBS extension coursing through the neck and terminating in the left chest wall. (a) There is discontinuity in the wiring at the level of the left mastoid process. (b and c) The DBS lead and extension are coiled in the extracranial soft tissues.

complication. Use of the newer connectors, combined with proper placement under the scalp and meticulous galea closure work, will decrease the risk of skin erosion.[52,72] Larger neurostimulators may also be more likely to cause skin erosions. Skin erosions may also occur because of extremely tight suturing over the device, or in those elderly patients with thin, frail skin.

Prevention

Erosions of the skin above the neurostimulator can be prevented by implanting the lead connector or neurostimulator into a deeper tissue plane and using one tunnel for each neurostimulator.[80] Skin above the DBS system should be checked at each visit so that problems that may cause skin erosion can be identified and treated early.

Troubleshooting

If the erosion occurs over the connector, it can be relocated into a trough drilled in the skull. If the erosion occurs over the neurostimulator, a complete revision of the device is required, moving it to a deeper plane if necessary.[48,81] If the erosion occurs over the burr hole and no infection was found, a skin revision may be sufficient. Sometimes a revision is needed to replace the burr-hole ring and cap assembly using bone cement or methacrylate and a ligature or plate to lessen pressure on the incision and help closure of the wound.

DBS lead or wire break (Figure 9.7)

Most lead or wire breaks occur between the extension cable and the DBS brain lead, which is usually located below the mastoid process.[82,83] Head turning can also move the DBS lead connector and can break the system circuit. The incidence of lead or wire break has been reported to be 5.1%.[48] Some patients may feel an "electric shock" sensation that is worsened by pressing on the area of the lead. Impulse control disorders such as trichotillomania[84] and twiddler syndrome have been reported to cause DBS lead or wire fractures.[85–88] In twiddler syndrome, the patient deliberately or subconsciously spins the neurostimulator in the chest region. When the patient spins the neurostimulator, the lead is shortened and an open circuit occurs, causing an electrical sensation in the patient's body. Alternatively this may also result in a lead fracture.

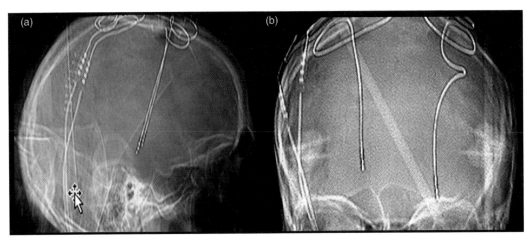

Figure 9.8 Lead migration in a patient with globus pallidus internus deep brain stimulation (GPi DBS). Plain skull X-ray lateral (a) and AP (b) showing lead migration status post GPi DBS in a patient with generalized torsion dystonia who developed worsening of symptoms that were previously controlled by DBS. The left lead had moved 10.4 mm downward and the right lead had moved 4.7 mm upward.

Prevention

To prevent lead fracture, the DBS lead connector should be mounted on the skull (parietal subgalea) and not in the neck.

Troubleshooting

Impedances and associated current drain should be checked. A high impedance and low current drain usually indicates a break or open circuit. A low impedance and high current drain usually indicates a short circuit.[89] In a twiddler patient, it is necessary to create a new suitably sized pocket under the pectoralis muscle fascia (usually on the contralateral side), suture the device to the muscle, and use a Parsonnet pouch to prevent electrode or wire break.[86,90]

Lead migration (Figure 9.8)

Lead migration, a rare event, usually occurs when fixation of the lead to the skull is inadequate.[72,83] In dystonia, the lead mostly shifts downward due to head movement, dragging the extension cable and neurostimulator upward.[91] Another potential cause of lead migration is skull growth in children.[44]

Prevention

Lead migration can be prevented by carefully securing the DBS lead and anchoring the lead using the burr-hole ring and cap in the subgaleal space. If using a titanium microplate[92] be sure not to crush the lead under it. After the lead is anchored, make a wide lead wire loop around the cap to reduce traction when

there is pulling of the system.[91] Perform intraoperative fluoroscopy to make sure the lead is in the correct location before closing the scalp incision.

Troubleshooting

1. Verify lead position by performing serial postoperative scans, especially in patients with waning clinical benefit.
2. Determine whether there is a movement of the lead(s).
3. If there is dorsal displacement, compensate with reprogramming (using the deepest/ventral electrode for reprogramming).
4. Consider another surgery for repositioning and replacement of the DBS lead if clinical benefit cannot be recaptured.

Neurostimulator malfunction (Figure 9.9)

Most neurostimulator malfunctions occurred with the early neurostimulator model (Itrel II, Medtronic, Inc.) and are now uncommon. Patients had complained of shocking sensations or intermittent stimulation around the neurostimulator site.[72]

Prevention

During follow-up visits, the clinician needs to verify proper functioning of the device.

Neurostimulator migration

Neurostimulator migration results mainly from a change in subcutaneous position of the device and

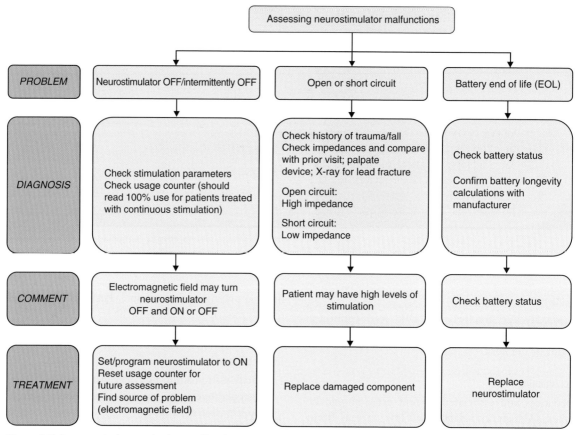

Figure 9.9 Assessment of neurostimulator malfunction.

may be due to inadequate securing of the device during implantation or obesity of the patient. Compulsive behavior (twiddler syndrome) may increase the risk of device migration and lead or extension fracture.[88]

Prevention

Migration can be prevented in many cases by suturing the neurostimulator under the underlying fascia below the pectoralis muscle using a polyester pouch.

Troubleshooting

Verify the diagnosis by visualizing the neurostimulator with a "shunt series" X-ray examination. Problems can be managed by surgical revision.

Pain/discomfort over the neurostimulator

Pain/discomfort over the neurostimulator is mostly found in thin patients whose lead-extension path has

one tissue tunnel for both lead extensions (36%), rather than in those with a single tunnel for each lead extension (11%).[80]

Prevention

Consider implantation of the neurostimulator in the abdominal region for thin patients.[80] In our own experience, we have not found this approach of abdominal implantation to be helpful, and we usually opt for a more conservative approach that may also include exercises of the neck region.

Troubleshooting

Capsaicin topical cream 0.025% or 0.075%[47] can be applied 4 times a day over the neurostimulator region to reduce pain. Neurostimulator repositioning may be necessary if capsaicin treatment fails to relieve the pain/discomfort.

Management of stimulation-related issues

Stimulation-related issues usually result from the spread of electrical current into brain regions other than the region intended for stimulation and from suboptimal lead placement. The clinician programming the DBS system should bear in mind that stimulation using an appropriately placed DBS lead should not produce stimulation-induced adverse effects at low to medium levels of stimulation but is expected to produce stimulation-related adverse effects at medium to high levels of stimulation. For example, in DBS of the thalamic Vim nucleus, stimulation can produce paresthesia, dysarthria, muscle contraction, and postural instability, depending on the levels of stimulation. With DBS of the STN, patients may experience dysarthria, tonic muscle contraction, dyskinesia, paresthesia, and diplopia. In response to DBS of the GPi, there may be hypophonia, dysarthria, tonic muscle contraction, paresthesia, and visual phosphenes. Poorly placed DBS leads result in adverse effects at stimulation levels lower than that required for clinical benefit. Stimulation-related adverse effects are reversible and may be avoided in many cases by adjusting stimulation parameters.

> Stimulation using an appropriately placed DBS lead should not produce stimulation-induced adverse effects at low to medium levels of stimulation but is expected to produce stimulation-related adverse effects at medium to high levels of stimulation.

> A poorly placed DBS lead either produces stimulation-related adverse effects at relatively low levels of stimulation or does not produce any effects, beneficial or adverse, at relatively high levels of stimulation.

Troubleshooting

Test stimulation through each electrode on the DBS lead should be performed in a monopolar configuration, with gradual escalation of stimulation amplitude; amplitude thresholds for the emergence of adverse effects should be explored and documented. If stimulation-related adverse effects occur outside the expected range (that is, at relatively low levels of stimulation) or not at all, imaging should be performed (preferably with brain MRI following the safety precautions provided by the device manufacturer or with

CT scan fused to the preoperative MRI). This will usually help to verify if the DBS lead is in an acceptable position, and it can help in choosing the best electrode on the DBS lead for therapeutic stimulation. If the DBS lead is found to be in an inappropriate location, stereotactic surgical repositioning may be required.

Problems specific to thalamic Vim DBS (Figure 9.10)

Paresthesia

Paresthesia is defined as an abnormal sensation of the skin, such as numbness, tingling, pricking, or burning. As stimulation level is increased, transient paresthesia may occur, usually disappearing within a few seconds. At higher levels of stimulation, up to 10% of patients will experience persistent paresthesia.[93] This effect is due to electrical current from the active electrode(s) stimulating the ventralis caudalis (Vc) nucleus of the thalamus or the lemniscal fibers.[94]

Troubleshooting

Persistence of paresthesia can be managed by reprogramming the device (lowering the amplitude or pulse width, or by changing the electrode configuration). If reprogramming fails to provide the patient with adequate tremor control in the absence of persistent, bothersome paresthesia, repositioning of the DBS lead should be considered.[95]

Muscle contraction

Muscle contraction occurs when stimulation spreads into the internal capsule.[96] The contracting muscles correspond to the region of the capsular homunculus.

Troubleshooting

Muscle contraction can be diminished by reducing the stimulation level or by changing the electrode configuration.[97]

If reprogramming fails to provide the patient with adequate tremor control in the absence of persistent muscle contraction, repositioning of the DBS lead should be considered.[95]

Dysarthria

Approximately 5–25% of patients will experience stimulation-induced dysarthria with bilateral Vim DBS.[98–100] Dysarthria may be caused by stimulation current spread to the internal capsule/

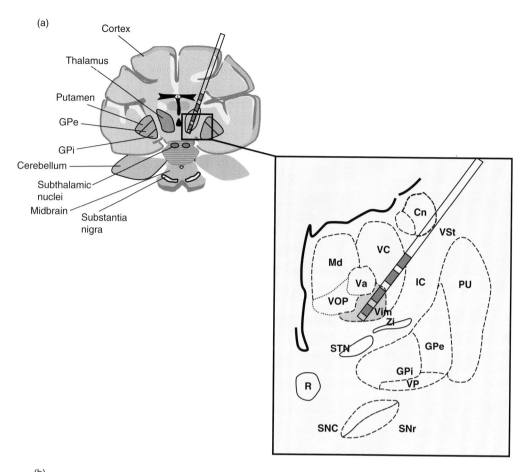

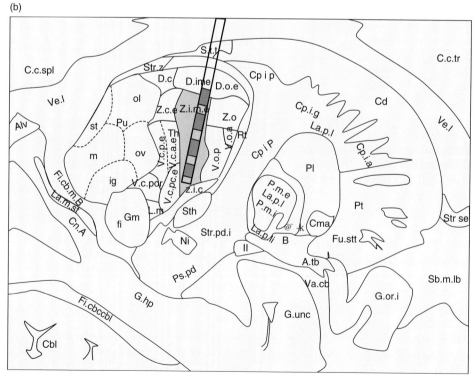

Figure 9.10 Thalamic ventral intermedius (Vim) nucleus deep brain stimulation (DBS) lead location in coronal (a) and sagittal (b) planes.

corticobulbar fibers, since the Vim is anatomically close to internal capsule.[97,101]

Patients with dysarthria following Vim DBS should be examined in two conditions: "on" stimulation and "off" stimulation. Dysarthria due to stimulation will get worse when stimulation is "on." This can be treated by decreasing the stimulation parameters or changing the configuration of electrodes, especially to a bipolar montage. If the DBS lead was placed too lateral, the stimulation will influence corticobulbar fibers and cause dysarthria at a level of stimulation that is insufficient to control tremor. This problem can be managed by repositioning the DBS lead, although many patients opt to accept the presence of some dysarthria in exchange for tremor control (and can use their patient programmer to adjust stimulation levels to optimize either tremor control or clarity of speech, depending on their circumstances).

Postural instability/ataxia (Figure 9.11)

Postural instability and other problems with balance have been reported following Vim DBS, with an incidence of approximately 3–7%.[95] These problems seem to be associated with bilateral stimulation. The symptoms may reverse in some cases with stimulation parameter changes,[98,100–104] usually reductions in amplitude or pulse width, or switching to bipolar configuration.

Problems specific to STN DBS (Figures 9.12 and 9.13)

Dyskinesia/hemiballismus

Stimulation-induced dyskinesia with STN DBS appears to be a sign of a well-located DBS lead. Dyskinesia may occur minutes to hours after stimulation is initiated or increased, requiring that the clinician programmer be patient while evaluating the subject and, if possible, observe them after some time has passed. Controlling dyskinesia is best accomplished by balancing stimulation parameters and dopaminergic medication.[95] Often, reduction of medications is the most effective treatment.

Paresthesia

Paresthesia usually occurs as a result of stimulation current spread to the medial lemniscus, which passes ventroposteriorly to the STN. In most instances these paresthesiae are transient, rapidly disappearing. Persistent paresthesia may indicate that the DBS lead is located too deep, posterior, and medial. Adjusting the stimulation parameters or electrode configuration usually resolves this problem.[95]

Muscle contraction

Muscle contraction in STN stimulation is due to current spread into the internal capsule.[95,96] The muscles that contract correspond to the region of the capsular homunculus.[97]

Troubleshooting

Muscle contraction can be diminished by reducing the stimulation level to be below the threshold by which this effect occurs or by changing the electrode configuration. If reprogramming fails to resolve this problem, repositioning of the DBS lead should be considered.[95,97]

Dysarthria/dysphonia/hypophonia

The prevalence of impaired speech after STN DBS ranges from 4 to 17%,[6,105–107] and this impairment typically occurs after bilateral STN DBS. Most studies assume that speech impairment is due to current spread to internal capsule and corticobulbar fibers,[97,101,108] but it may be also related to the progression of PD.

Troubleshooting

For speech problems after STN DBS, adjust and optimize stimulation parameters and consider the effects of left versus right stimulation and the effects of medications. Speech therapy may be helpful, and in severe situations patients may need to temporarily turn off one stimulator (usually the left) when speaking.[109–111]

Gait impairment/postural instability

Gait impairment and postural instability are improved after STN DBS,[112] but will often worsen after 5 years due to the progression of PD.[6,106,113]

Troubleshooting

Balancing the stimulation parameters, dopaminergic medication, and occupational/physiotherapy seems to be helpful in improving gait and postural impairment in patients with PD. In the case of stimulation-induced postural instability with truncal ataxia, suboptimal lead location is usually the cause, resulting in stimulation current spread to the red nucleus or cerebellar fibers.[114] This complication can be managed by revision of the DBS lead.

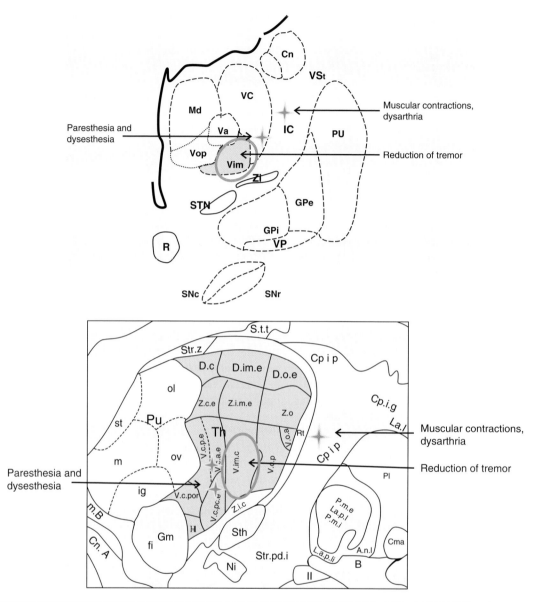

CLINICAL EFFECT	ELECTRODE LOCATION
Paresthesia at low amplitude of stimulation	Potentially too posterior
Dysarthria at low amplitude of stimulation	Potentially too lateral/posteromedial
Tonic contraction at low amplitude of stimulation	Potentially too lateral
No adverse or beneficial effects at high amplitude of stimulation	Potentially too superior or anterior

Figure 9.11 Thalamic ventral intermedius (Vim) nucleus deep brain stimulation (DBS): stimulation-induced effects. Cn, caudate nucleus; GPe, globus pallidus externa; GPi, globus pallidus interna; IC, internal capsule; Md, nucleus mediodorsal thalamus; Pu, putamen; R, red nucleus; SNc, subtantia nigra pars compacta; SNr, substantia nigra pars reticulata; STN, subthalamic nucleus; Va, nucleus ventral anterior thalamus; Vc, nucleus ventrocaudal thalamus; Vim, nucleus ventral intermedius thalamus; VP, visual pathway/optic tract; Vop, nucleus ventral oral posterior thalamus; VSt, ventral striatum; Zi, zona inserta.

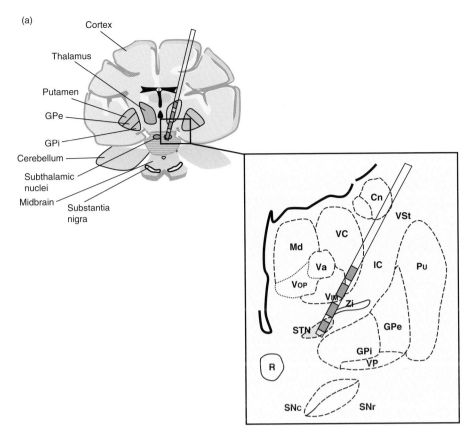

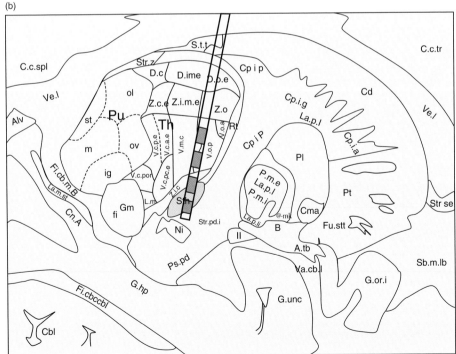

Figure 9.12 Subthalamic nucleus deep brain stimulation (STN DBS) lead location in coronal (a) and sagittal (b) planes. Cn, caudate nucleus; GPe, globus pallidus externa; GPi, globus pallidus interna; IC, internal capsule; Md, nucleus mediodorsal thalamus; Pu, putamen; R, red nucleus; SNc, subtantia nigra pars compacta; SNr, substantia nigra pars reticulata; STN, subthalamic nucleus; Va, nucleus ventral anterior thalamus; Vc, nucleus ventrocaudal thalamus; Vim, nucleus ventral intermedius thalamus; VP, visual pathway/optic tract; Vop, nucleus ventral oral posterior thalamus; VSt, ventral striatum; Zi, zona inserta.

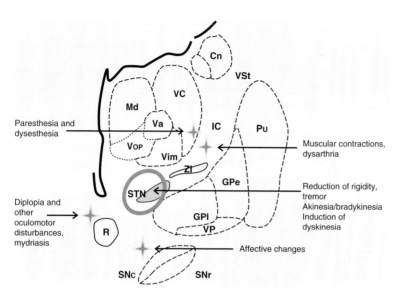

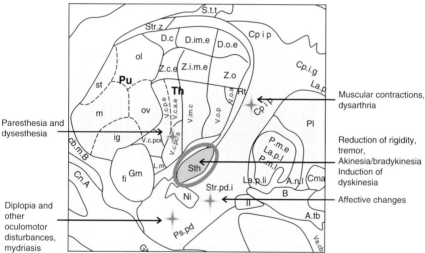

CLINICAL EFFECT	ELECTRODE LOCATION
Dyskinesia	In optimal location
Paresthesia at low amplitude of stimulation	Potentially too posterior or medial
Tonic muscle contraction at low amplitude of stimulation	Potentially too lateral or too anterior
Dysarthria at low amplitude of stimulation	Potentially too lateral or too anterior
Diplopia at low amplitude of stimulation	Usually too anteromedial
Mood change at low amplitude of stimulation	Potentially too inferior or medial
No adverse or beneficial effects at high amplitude of stimulation	Potentially too superior or anterior

Figure 9.13 Subthalamic nucleus deep brain stimulation (STN DBS): stimulation-induced effects. Cn, caudate nucleus; GPe, globus pallidus externa; GPi, globus pallidus interna; IC, internal capsule; Md, nucleus mediodorsal thalamus; Pu, putamen; R, red nucleus; SNc, subtantia nigra pars compacta; SNr, substantia nigra pars reticulata; STN, subthalamic nucleus; Va, nucleus ventral anterior thalamus; Vc, nucleus ventrocaudal thalamus; Vim, nucleus ventral intermedius thalamus; VP, visual pathway/optic tract; Vop, nucleus ventral oral posterior thalamus; VSt, ventral striatum; Zi, zona inserta.

Abnormal eye movements/diplopia

Double vision (diplopia) is usually due to stimulation of supranuclear oculomotor fibers below or medial to the STN, causing disconjugate eye movement. Patients may experience dizziness when viewing images displaced horizontally, vertically, or diagonally.

Troubleshooting

Most of the disconjugate eye movements after DBS are transient, due to habituation. If symptoms persist after the stimulation parameters and electrode configuration are optimized, revision of the lead is required.[95]

Apraxia of eyelid opening

Apraxia of eyelid opening (ALO) is a condition in which patients who have otherwise normal eyelids have difficulty opening the eyelids and experience involuntary closure of the eyes. It may occur following STN stimulation in patients who obtain good motor symptom improvement with DBS.[97,115] This adverse event is infrequent, occurring with an incidence of approximately 5%.[62] The mechanism of ALO is not well understood, and it can occur with relatively low stimulation parameters. Adjustment of the stimulation parameters may or may not be of benefit.

Troubleshooting

Most ALO patients are successfully treated by injection of botulinum toxin in both eyelid regions,[115] or by reprogramming the device to deliver stimulation using a different electrode configuration. When botulinum toxin is used, the injections are usually given at the pars palpebralis of the orbicularis oculi muscle and are required to be repeated every three to six months. These injections carry minimal risk of transient adverse effects such as hematoma, double vision, dryness of the eyes, or ptosis.[116]

Neuropsychiatric complications (Figure 9.14)

Neuropsychiatric complications vary greatly in manifestation. These complications have been increasingly documented following DBS surgery. Some of the more common neuropsychiatric conditions that have been found after DBS surgery are transient confusion, anxiety, apathy, hypomania, emotional instability, depression, suicidal tendencies, psychosis/hallucination, and compulsive or impulsive behavior.[117] A psychiatric referral may be needed to help evaluate and treat the patient.

Anxiety or emotional reactivity is the most common non-motor symptom in PD. It occurs in 75% of patients pre- and postoperatively.[118,119] Anxiety frequently occurs in patients who suffer from depression, panic attacks, and phobia. A trial of a benzodiazepine, cognitive behavioral therapy (CBT), and exposure therapy may help.

Transient confusion has been reported to occur in 1–36% of patients in the immediate postoperative phase.[6,69,70,120] Since it usually improves with time, no immediate treatment is needed.

Apathy also occurs, with a reported approximate incidence of 12–25% after STN DBS therapy.[6] It is sometimes brought about by depression associated with the reduction of dopaminergic medication that often occurs when motor symptoms are improved by DBS; increasing the dose of levodopa may therefore help to alleviate the apathy. The patient should be assessed for depression or mood disorder and given antidepressants if needed. Depression itself occurs in 1.5–25% of patients following STN DBS treatment.[6,70,121–123] It can be caused by many factors, such as the natural history of PD itself, dopaminergic medication withdrawal, stimulation current spread to the medial limbic system, and psychosocial factors like unrealistic patient expectations and poor family support. It is managed by treating the underlying cause of the depression by adjusting levodopa medication, giving antidepressant medications, modifying the stimulation parameters, and consulting with a psychiatrist.[117]

Hypomania occurs in 4–15% of patients post DBS surgery.[70,121] Troubleshoot postoperative hypomania by adjusting the dose of levodopa and giving a trial of antidepressants and mood stabilizers. A cholinesterase inhibitor may be given if cognitive impairment is present, and CBT may also be beneficial. In some cases moving the active stimulation electrode ventrally has improved the situation.

Prevalence of suicide attempts after DBS varies from 0.5% to 2.9%.[6,117,119,124,125] Depression, hypomania/mania, and psychotic symptoms should be evaluated, and patients exhibiting the behaviors and symptoms of these neuropsychiatric conditions need to be admitted and referred to a psychiatrist for proper management.

Psychosis (11%) and transient hallucination (16%) have also been reported in association with DBS.[35] The physician should consider admitting the patient to adjust dopaminergic medication and stimulation

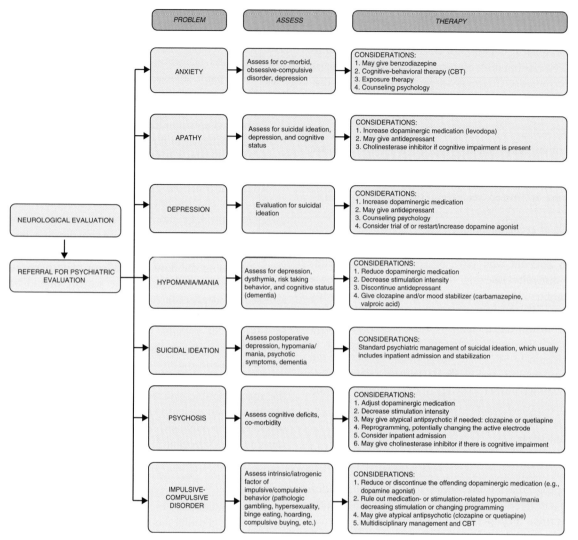

Figure 9.14 Management of neuropsychiatric complications.

parameters. An atypical antipsychotic may be given to treat psychosis.

Impulsive-compulsive disorder (e.g., pathological gambling, hypersexuality, binge eating, compulsive shopping, and hoarding) may be due to underlying dopamine dysregulation. It can be addressed in select cases by decreasing or discontinuing dopaminergic medication, adjusting DBS parameters, or giving atypical antipsychotics.

Cardiovascular reflexes

Based on the pathophysiological circuitry model of basal ganglia function in PD, there is an increased excitatory output from the STN that may result in an increased inhibitory output from the thalamus.[126] This is hypothesized to reduce the compensatory tachycardic response to postural changes required to prevent symptomatic orthostasis,[127] and the effects of DBS are thought to potentially impact autonomic function.

An observation by Sauleau et al.,[128] who directly monitored for intraoperative autonomic changes in patients who underwent STN DBS for PD, showed that 88% of patients have tachycardia within seconds after stimulation, followed by a hypertension interval in approximately 1 minute. This effect is temporary and will return to normal a few minutes following discontinuation of DBS.[129] Some studies suggest that

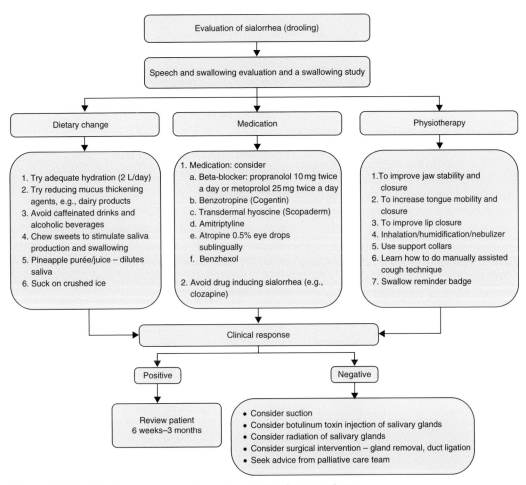

Figure 9.15 Algorithm for management of sialorrhea post deep brain stimulation.

tachycardia may persist for six months after DBS treatment with high frequency stimulation[130] and disappear after one year.[129] The long-term clinical significance of transient tachycardia and hypertension is still unknown.

Troubleshooting

Close monitoring of blood pressure and pulse rate after DBS is essential. Fluctuations in blood pressure or cardiovascular function can be managed medically. Antihypertensive medications may need to be reduced in dose and hydration increased.

Sialorrhea

Increasing sialorrhea as an adverse effect of STN DBS has been reported.[118,131] This issue may also be complicated by the coexistence of worsening in cognitive function, which may contribute to a reduced control

of secretions. Increased drooling has been reported in patients who underwent STN DBS.[132] It is unclear whether this is an effect of DBS or if there are other factors, such as natural progression of disease or modification of medication regimens, that may have influenced this outcome.

Troubleshooting

Most practitioners use anticholinergics and/or botulinum toxin in a case by case manner (Figure 9.15).

Dysphagia

Dysphagia has been reported in 4–8% of patients after STN DBS.[107,122,133] It remains unclear whether this results directly from the DBS or reflects disease progression and involvement of non-dopaminergic pathways. A comparison of swallowing function before and after STN DBS found no significant difference.[112]

This finding is consistent with the presence of a dopaminergically mediated component to swallowing. In some cases, however, DBS may influence corticospinal and corticobulbar fibers and worsen swallowing.

Troubleshooting

A swallowing study needs to be performed in both "on" and "off" stimualtion conditions if DBS-related swallowing problems are suspected. Reprogramming DBS parameters and medication adjustment may benefit some patients. A referral to a nutritionist may be helpful for dietary evaluation and adjustment.

Hypersexuality

The prevalence of hypersexuality in PD is estimated at 2.4%.[134] Most studies[112,135–137] report that men treated with STN DBS have an increased frequency, increased satisfaction, and decreased avoidance of sexual activity, especially those younger than 60 years of age; no significant change was found in sexual functioning for women. The mechanism for excessive sexual excitement after DBS is currently unknown.

Troubleshooting

Reducing dopaminergic medications[138] and/or reprogramming DBS parameters may be beneficial. Atypical antipsychotic medication[139] can be used in select cases. Donepezil hydrochloride also may aid in some cases of compulsive hypersexuality.[140]

Weight gain

Weight gain is common after DBS at the STN or GPi targets. It occurs at an incidence of 6–100% after STN DBS[6,107,135] and 26–96% after GPi DBS.[141] There have been no reports regarding weight gain after Vim DBS. Most patients will have weight gain of approximately 9.3–9.7 kg and an increase in body mass index by 4.7 kg/m^2 1 year post STN DBS treatment.[142,143]

There are several explanations for weight gain following STN DBS: (1) Changes in dopaminergic medications may also increase the drive for food intake. (2) There is decreased energy expenditure due to less motor fluctuation and dyskinesia. (3) Normalization of energy metabolism following STN implantation may favor body weight gain (men gained mass, while women gained fat).[144] (4) Spread of electrical current into non-motor regions, such as the hypothalamus, can induce changes in eating behavior. (5) Other factors, such as changes in living style and physical activities, may be involved.

Troubleshooting

Nutritional counseling to prevent rapid and excessive weight gain, as well as the initiation of an exercise program, can be useful.

Problems specific to GPi DBS (Figures 9.16 and 9.17)
Muscle contraction

Muscle contraction with GPi DBS results from stimulation current spread into the internal capsule.[96] The internal capsule is located posteriorly and medially from GPi. Clinicians need to be very careful to distinguish between tonic muscle contraction and dystonia, which can be challenging.

Troubleshooting

During DBS programming, the clinician needs to differentiate dystonia from capsular effects (that is, an effect caused by spread of the stimulation into the fibers of the internal capsule). If a capsular effect is elicited, reprogramming at lower amplitude or pulse width or changing the electrode configuration may be performed. If low-threshold capsular responses prevent adequate stimulation, then DBS lead revision may be considered.

Dysarthria/hypophonia

Dysarthria/hypophonia with GPi DBS is rare, although its occurrence has been reported.[70,145] Administering speech and swallowing examinations both on and off stimulation may help in the diagnosis.

Troubleshooting

Testing different DBS parameters and medication combinations, along with speech therapy, may help improve dysarthria.[109–112]

Visual phenomena

During intraoperative microelectrode recording, identification of the optic tract is used to help determine the ventral border of GPi.[146] If the DBS lead is implanted near the optic tract and electrical current spreads to the optic tract region, the patient will report seeing sparkles of light (phosphenes). Homonymus quadrantanopsia can occur after GPi DBS

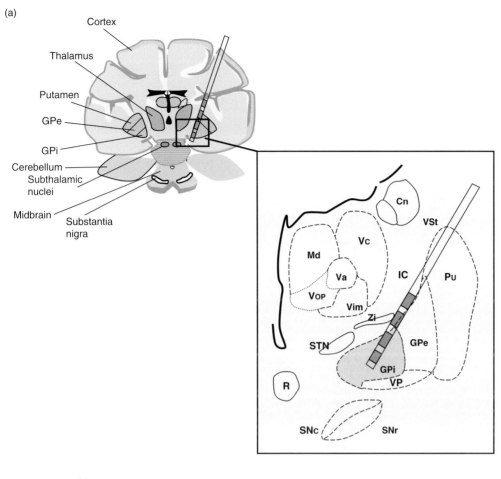

(a)

Cortex
Thalamus
Putamen
GPe
GPi
Cerebellum
Subthalamic
nuclei
Midbrain
Substantia
nigra

Cn
VSt
Vc
Md
Va
IC
Pu
Vop
Vim
Zi
STN
GPe
R
GPi
VP
SNc
SNr

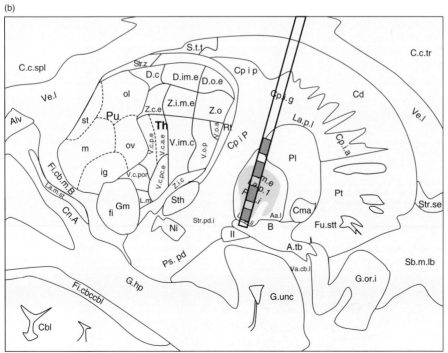

(b)

C.c.spl
S.t.t
Cp i p
C.c.tr
Str.z
Ve.l
D.c
D.im.e
D.o.e
Cp.i.g
Cd
Alv
ol
Z.i.m.e
Z.o
La.p.l
Ve.l
Z.c.e
st
Pu
Th
V.o.a
Rt
Cp.i.a
m
ov
V.c.p.e
V.im.c
V.o.p
Cp i P
Pl
Pt
ig
V.c.por
V.c.pc.e
Z.i.c
La.m.e
Str.se
Fi.cb.m.B
L.m
La.o.1
La.m.st
Gm
Sth
Cma
Fu.stt
Cn.A
fi
Ni
Str.pd.i
Aa.l
B
Sb.m.lb
ll
A.tb
Ps. pd
Va.cb.l
G.or.i
G.hp
G.unc
Fi.cbccbl
Cbl

117

Figure 9.16 Globus pallidus internus deep brain stimulation (GPi DBS) lead location in coronal (a) and sagittal (b) planes.

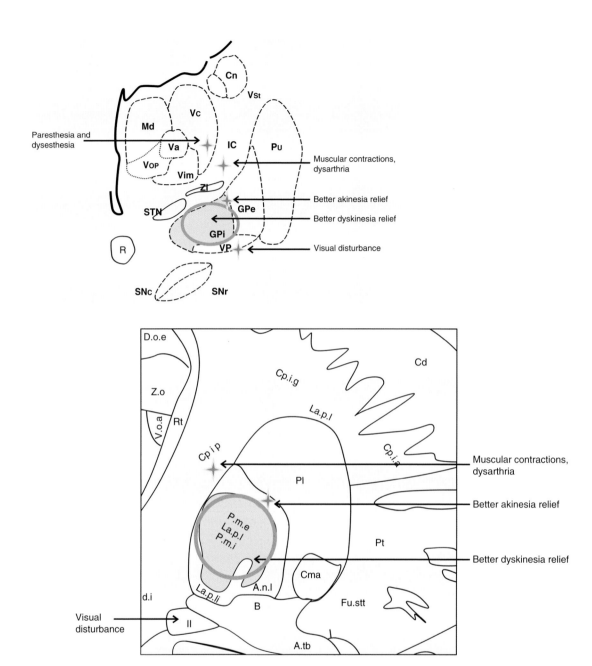

CLINICAL EFFECT	ELECTRODE LOCATION
Dysarthria at low amplitude of stimulation	Potentially too posteromedial
Tonic muscle contraction at low amplitude of stimulation	Potentially too posteromedial
Visual phenomena at low amplitude of stimulation	Close to optic pathways
No adverse or beneficial effects at high amplitude of stimulation	Potentially too superior, anterior, or lateral

Figure 9.17 Globus pallidus internus deep brain stimulation (GPi DBS): stimulation-induced effects. Cn, caudate nucleus; GPe, globus pallidus externa; GPi, globus pallidus interna; IC, internal capsule; Md, nucleus mediodorsal thalamus; Pu, putamen; R, red nucleus; SNc, subtantia nigra pars compacta; SNr, substantia nigra pars reticulata; STN, subthalamic nucleus; Va, nucleus ventral anterior thalamus; Vc, nucleus ventrocaudal thalamus; Vim, nucleus ventral intermedius thalamus; VP, visual pathway/optic tract; Vop, nucleus ventral oral posterior thalamus; VSt, ventral striatum; Zi, zona inserta.

from a lesion of the optic tract, but this is rare in DBS and is more common in pallidotomy.[147]

Troubleshooting

Persistence of phosphenes can be managed by using a more dorsal electrode for stimulation or by repositioning the DBS lead if stimulation parameter adjustment fails to resolve this problem.[95]

Troubleshooting other DBS-related issues

Disease progression

Worsening of symptoms may occur over time, even when the patient has been deriving benefit from DBS for years. This may simply signify progression of the disease and not device failure.

Troubleshooting

Perform imaging studies to determine if there has been migration of the DBS lead (an uncommon occurrence). Re-examine the patient using standardized rating scales. For patients with PD, assessment of the UPDRS examination while "off" medication and "off" stimulation and then again while "on" medication and "off" stimulation will identify levodopa-responsive symptoms. If the symptom does not improve with levodopa, then it is also unlikely to respond to changes in DBS programming or lead placement (the notable exception being tremor).[31,44]

Poor DBS candidate/lack of evaluation by a multidisciplinary team

Ideally, a multidisciplinary team should be involved in selecting patients for treatment with DBS.[44,148,149]

This team consists of a movement disorder-trained neurologist and neurosurgeon, nurse, physician assistant, psychiatrist, neuropsychologist, occupational therapist, nutritionist, speech pathologist, social worker, a financial counselor, and home care case manager. Each team member independently assesses the patient, and the team then gathers together to review and discuss their findings in a team meeting. In the meeting, the multidisciplinary team will determine whether the patients are qualified for DBS surgery or not.

Several criteria need to be fulfilled to make the patients eligible for treatment with DBS. For those with PD, patients need to have a clear diagnosis of idiopathic PD (preferably diagnosed by a movement disorder specialist[150]). They should not have atypical parkinsonian features. Patients should demonstrate a clear (even if only brief) response to dopaminergic medication, with improvement in the UPDRS motor score of at least 30% between the off- and on-medication states.[151] There should be absence of active psychiatric illness and little or no cognitive impairment. Other considerations, such as age, general health, and patient expectations, should also be reviewed (Table 9.5).

A general practitioner/neurologist can use a screening tool, the Florida Surgical Questionnaire for Parkinson's Disease (FLASQ-PD),[152] to help identify and triage patients with PD who are being considered for treatment with DBS. This questionnaire consists of five domains: (1) criteria for diagnosing PD; (2) eight potential contraindications/red flags to DBS surgery (e.g., supranuclear palsy, dementia, psychosis, unresponsive to levodopa, etc.); (3) patient characteristics; (4) favorable/unfavorable symptoms (e.g., depression, cognitive status, etc.); and (5) medication trials. This screening can be administered in approximately 10–15 minutes. The best candidates for DBS surgery usually score 25 or greater and have no "red flags."

Dystonia and ET patients should be evaluated in a similar manner.

Unrealistic patient expectations/failure to achieve patient expectations

Treatment with DBS can suppress motor signs and symptoms, improve functional abilities, and enhance quality of life – but it is not a cure for movement disorders. Results of DBS surgery may vary from patient to patient. Sometimes optimal results from stimulation may require months to years to be achieved. The clinician should discuss this with the patient and his/her family to ensure reasonable expectations.[31]

Prevention

Ask the patient to write his/her expectations about the outcomes from DBS and document this in the chart prior to surgery. These notes can be referred back to after the surgery for better outcome assessment. Good preoperative counseling and education before DBS surgery should be mandatory.[31,44] Useful adjuncts include the National Parkinson Foundation (NPF) booklet[153] and a mnemonic device developed by Okun and Foote (Figure 9.18).[43]

Table 9.5 Favorable or unfavorable characteristics for deep brain stimulation candidates[44]

Diagnosis	Ideal characteristics for DBS	Potentially unfavorable characteristics for DBS
Parkinson's disease	• Significant "on/off" fluctuations, despite best medical treatment • Dyskinesia • Disabling tremor • PD symptoms are clearly medication-responsive (e.g., significant improvement in the UPDRS motor scores in the "on" state compared to the "off" state) • Non-fixed dystonia	• Difficult to control hallucinations • Moderate to severe cognitive problems • Presence of multiple "primitive" reflexes • Incontinence of bowel and bladder • Gait and balance impairment that are not responsive to dopaminergic treatment • Active, untreated psychiatric issues • Underlying severe psychiatric diagnosis • Structural abnormality on brain imaging (beyond mild atrophy, mild white matter hyperintensities, or calcifications) • Underlying severe medical co-morbidity
Dystonia	• Diagnosis of: Primary generalized dystonia • Cervical dystonia • Tardive dystonia syndromes • Dystonia is mobile (i.e., not fixed)	• Presence of contractures • Moderate to severe cognitive problems • Presence of significant bony deformities • Secondary etiologies/other dystonias (except tardive dystonia) • Presence of multiple primitive reflexes • Incontinence of bowel and bladder • Active, untreated psychiatric issues • Underlying severe psychiatric diagnosis • Structural abnormality on brain imaging • Underlying severe medical co-morbidity • Able to adequately control symptoms with pharmacological treatment
Essential tremor	• Disabling postural/action tremor • Medication refractory	• Moderate to severe cognitive problems • Presence of severe limb ataxia along with the essential tremor • Presence of severe gait ataxia • Presence of multiple primitive reflexes • Incontinence of bowel and bladder • Active, untreated psychiatric issues • Underlying severe psychiatric diagnosis Structural abnormality on brain imaging • Underlying severe medical co-morbidity • Still able to adequately control symptoms with pharmacological treatment

Notes: DBS, deep brain stimulation; PD, Parkinson's disease; UPDRS, Unified Parkinson's Disease Rating Scale.

Troubleshooting

Have the patient keep a diary to assess the improvements or deterioration in his or her symptoms.

Poor access to DBS programming

DBS management usually requires multiple visits. Patients usually come every month or two in the first six months to be assessed,[31] and then every three to six months thereafter. Follow up may become troublesome for those who live far from an experienced center.

Prevention

The clinician should explain the importance of patient commitment, follow up, and family support prior to performing the surgery. Ablative surgery may be the best option for patients who live in a remote area (especially since it requires less follow up).[44]

DBS IS NOT A CURE

BILATERAL DBS IS OFTEN REQUIRED TO IMPROVE GAIT

SMOOTHES OUT ON/OFF FLUCTUATIONS

IMPROVES TREMOR, RIGIDITY, BRADYKINESIA, AND DYSKINESIA

NEVER IMPROVES SYMPTOMS THAT ARE UNRESPONSIVE TO LEVODOPA (EXCEPT TREMOR)

PROGRAMMING AND MEDICATION ADJUSTMENT ARE REQUIRED

DECREASES MEDICATIONS IN MANY, BUT NOT TO ZERO

DBS IN PD
mnemonic

Figure 9.18 University of Florida mnemonic device for Parkinson's disease patients considering deep brain stimulation. Modified and reprinted with permission from Michael S. Okun.[43]

Troubleshooting

The patient can be asked to follow up in the nearest local region that has a DBS practitioner for follow-up programming. It is important to assess the patient as many times as possible during the first six months to optimize DBS settings. Following this, most of the management should be medical.

Suboptimal DBS programming and medication adjustment

The neurologist and DBS programmer should work together to improve parkinsonian symptoms by balancing between medication and stimulation parameters.[44] In PD, medication mostly can be reduced, but in dystonia and ET they can often be stopped after surgery.

Several steps for finding the best balance between medication and DBS parameters include: (1) Perform a complete neurological examination and compare UPDRS motor scores in four conditions: "off" medication/"off" stimulation; "on" medication/"off" stimulation; "off" medication/ "on" stimulation; and "on" medication/"on" stimulation to determine stimulation and medication effects. (2) While the patient is off medication, test each electrode on the DBS lead in monopolar configuration to obtain amplitude thresholds for the

induction of beneficial and adverse effects and record these findings in the chart. (3) Optimize stimulation parameters. (4) Adjust medications once DBS programming is complete. (5) Repeat motor examinations using a rating scale to document improvement of symptoms. (6) Give motor diary to patients to identify fluctuations in motor symptoms. (7) Consider adjunctive therapies, such as physical therapy, occupational therapy, and speech therapy, to improve symptoms.

Approaches to medication adjustments for patients with PD include: (1) Use amantadine for patients with mild or moderate dyskinesia. (2) Administer an anticholinergic (trihexyphenidyl) or a high dose of levodopa plus a dopamine agonist for patients with medication-refractory tremor. (3) Administer carbidopa/levodopa immediate-release more frequently for on–off fluctuations and dyskinesia. (4) Use an apomorphine injection to rescue patients from sudden "off" periods. (5) In patients who have severe dyskinesia and on–off fluctuation, consider revision of medication to immediate release carbidopa/levodopa and addition of a dopamine agonist or catechol-O-methyltransferase (COMT) inhibitor. (6) For patients with nausea due to carbidopa/levodopa, add extra carbidopa to each dose.

121

Tolerance to DBS

In some patients, DBS can lose its effectiveness following an initial response. Detection of tolerance and habituation after DBS is difficult, and its mechanism is still unknown. It is most common in ET,[154] although it may occur in dystonia or PD. Generally, when tolerance occurs there may be 6–12 months of efficacy, followed by clinical symptom reoccurence.

Troubleshooting

Device malfunction, suboptimal lead location, and suboptimal DBS programming need to be ruled out. If tolerance is suspected, consideration can be given to DBS lead relocation, stimulating at a different brain target, or delivering stimulation on a cyclical basis.

Summary

Assessment of patients for DBS candidacy is best performed using a multidisciplinary team approach. Evaluation following DBS surgery includes motor function, quality of life, and other relevant clinical outcomes, including the neuropsychiatric status.

Problems encountered with DBS surgery can be divided into four main categories: (1) surgery-related; (2) device-related; (3) stimulation-related; and (4) other issues, including disease progression, poor DBS candidate/lack of the multidisciplinary team evaluation, unrealistic patient expectations/failure to achieve patient expectations, poor access to programming, improper programming and medication adjustment, and tolerance.

Most of the issues and complications stemming from DBS are treatable. Management of DBS failures should be tailored on a case by case basis.

Conclusions

Successful management of DBS entails an understanding of the indications and potential pitfalls of this therapy. Troubleshooting requires the use of a systematic approach to initial and follow-up device programming and patient management. This approach should include a detailed data gathering process prior to initiating therapy. The ability to troubleshoot problems in patients who do not achieve an optimal therapeutic response will be critical in attempting to convert DBS failures to successes. As with most procedures, efficiency of patient management will improve for each clinician with experience.

Acknowledgments

We would like to acknowledge the support of the National Parkinson Foundation Center of Excellence, the McKnight Brain Institute, and the Eric and Jennifer Scott Fund. Thanks to Kelly Byram for critical revision of the chapter.

References

1. Goetz CG, Fahn S, Martinez-Martin P, et al. Movement Disorder Society-sponsored revision of the Unified Parkinson's Disease Rating Scale (MDS-UPDRS): process, format, and clinimetric testing plan. *Mov Disord* 2007;**22**:41–7.

2. Defer GL, Widner H, Marie RM, Remy P, Levivier M. Core assessment program for surgical interventional therapies in Parkinson's disease (CAPSIT-PD). *Mov Disord* 1999;**14**:572–84.

3. Loher TJ, Burgunder JM, Pohle T, et al. Long-term pallidal deep brain stimulation in patients with advanced Parkinson disease: 1-year follow-up study. *J Neurosurg* 2002;**96**:844–53.

4. Germano IM, Gracies JM, Weisz DJ, et al. Unilateral stimulation of the subthalamic nucleus in Parkinson disease: a double-blind 12-month evaluation study. *J Neurosurg* 2004;**101**:36–42.

5. Weaver F, Follett K, Hur K, Ippolito D, Stern M. Deep brain stimulation in Parkinson disease: a metaanalysis of patient outcomes. *J Neurosurg* 2005;**103**:956–67.

6. Krack P, Batir A, Van Blercom N, et al. Five-year follow-up of bilateral stimulation of the subthalamic nucleus in advanced Parkinson's disease. *N Engl J Med* 2003;**349**:1925–34.

7. Koller WC, Lyons KE, Wilkinson SB, Troster AI, Pahwa R. Long-term safety and efficacy of unilateral deep brain stimulation of the thalamus in essential tremor. *Mov Disord* 2001;**16**:464–8.

8. Blomstedt P, Hariz GM, Hariz MI, Koskinen LO. Thalamic deep brain stimulation in the treatment of essential tremor: a long-term follow-up. *Br J Neurosurg* 2007;**21**:504–9.

9. Vickrey BG. Getting oriented to patient-oriented outcomes. *Neurology* 1999;**53**:662–3.

10. Guyatt GH, Bombardier C, Tugwell PX. Measuring disease-specific quality of life in clinical trials. *CMAJ* 1986;**134**:889–95.

11. Doward LC, McKenna SP. Defining patient-reported outcomes. *Value Health* 2004;7(Suppl 1):S4–8.

12. Ware JE, Jr., Sherbourne CD. The MOS 36-item short-form health survey (SF-36). I. Conceptual framework and item selection. *Med Care* 1992;**30**:473–83.

13. Hobson JP, Meara RJ. Is the SF-36 health survey questionnaire suitable as a self-report measure of the health status of older adults with Parkinson's disease? *Qual Life Res* 1997;**6**:213–16.

14. Hill S, Harries U, Popay J. Is the short form 36 (SF-36) suitable for routine health outcomes assessment in health care for older people? Evidence from preliminary work in community based health services in England. *J Epidemiol Community Health* 1996;**50**:94–8.

15. Hayes V, Morris J, Wolfe C, Morgan M. The SF-36 health survey questionnaire: is it suitable for use with older adults? *Age Ageing* 1995;**24**:120–5.

16. Hunt SM, McKenna SP, McEwen J, Williams J, Papp E. The Nottingham Health Profile: subjective health status and medical consultations. *Soc Sci Med [A]* 1981;**15**:221–9.

17. Kind P, Carr-Hill R. The Nottingham health profile: a useful tool for epidemiologists? *Soc Sci Med* 1987;**25**:905–10.

18. Bergner M, Bobbitt RA, Carter WB, Gilson BS. The Sickness Impact Profile: development and final revision of a health status measure. *Med Care* 1981;**19**:787–805.

19. Welsh M, McDermott MP, Holloway RG, et al. Development and testing of the Parkinson's disease quality of life scale. *Mov Disord* 2003;**18**:637–45.

20. Kuehler A, Henrich G, Schroeder U, et al. A novel quality of life instrument for deep brain stimulation in movement disorders. *J Neurol Neurosurg Psychiatry* 2003;**74**:1023–30.

21. Troster AI, Pahwa R, Fields JA, Tanner CM, Lyons KE. Quality of life in Essential Tremor Questionnaire (QUEST): development and initial validation. *Parkinsonism Relat Disord* 2005;**11**:367–73.

22. Mueller J, Skogseid IM, Benecke R, et al. Pallidal deep brain stimulation improves quality of life in segmental and generalized dystonia: results from a prospective, randomized sham-controlled trial. *Mov Disord* 2008;**23**:131–4.

23. Blahak C, Wohrle JC, Capelle HH, et al. Health-related quality of life in segmental dystonia is improved by bilateral pallidal stimulation. *J Neurol* 2008;**255**:178–82.

24. Halbig TD, Gruber D, Kopp UA, et al. Pallidal stimulation in dystonia: effects on cognition, mood, and quality of life. *J Neurol Neurosurg Psychiatry* 2005;**76**:1713–6.

25. Skogseid IM. Pallidal deep brain stimulation is effective, and improves quality of life in primary segmental and generalized dystonia. *Acta Neurol Scand Suppl* 2008;**188**:51–5.

26. Vingerhoets G, Lannoo E, van der Linden C, et al. Changes in quality of life following unilateral pallidal stimulation in Parkinson's disease. *J Psychosom Res* 1999;**46**:247–55.

27. Voon V, Saint-Cyr J, Lozano AM, et al. Psychiatric symptoms in patients with Parkinson disease presenting for deep brain stimulation surgery. *J Neurosurg* 2005;**103**:246–51.

28. Funkiewiez A, Ardouin C, Caputo E, et al. Long term effects of bilateral subthalamic nucleus stimulation on cognitive function, mood, and behaviour in Parkinson's disease. *J Neurol Neurosurg Psychiatry* 2004;**75**:834–9.

29. Castelli L, Perozzo P, Zibetti M, et al. Chronic deep brain stimulation of the subthalamic nucleus for Parkinson's disease: effects on cognition, mood, anxiety and personality traits. *Eur Neurol* 2006;**55**:136–44.

30. Mink JW, Walkup J, Frey KA, et al. Patient selection and assessment recommendations for deep brain stimulation in Tourette syndrome. *Mov Disord* 2006;**21**:1831–8.

31. Rodriguez RL, Fernandez HH, Haq I, Okun MS. Pearls in patient selection for deep brain stimulation. *Neurologist* 2007;**13**:253–60.

32. Contarino MF, Daniele A, Sibilia AH, et al. Cognitive outcome 5 years after bilateral chronic stimulation of subthalamic nucleus in patients with Parkinson's disease. *J Neurol Neurosurg Psychiatry* 2007;**78**:248–52.

33. Dujardin K, Defebvre L, Krystkowiak P, Blond S, Destee A. Influence of chronic bilateral stimulation of the subthalamic nucleus on cognitive function in Parkinson's disease. *J Neurol* 2001;**248**:603–11.

34. Moretti R, Torre P, Antonello RM, et al. Neuropsychological changes after subthalamic nucleus stimulation: a 12 month follow-up in nine patients with Parkinson's disease. *Parkinsonism Relat Disord* 2003;**10**:73–9.

35. Schupbach WM, Chastan N, Welter ML, et al. Stimulation of the subthalamic nucleus in Parkinson's disease: a 5 year follow up. *J Neurol Neurosurg Psychiatry* 2005;**76**:1640–4.

36. Schroeder U, Kuehler A, Haslinger B, et al. Subthalamic nucleus stimulation affects striato-anterior cingulate cortex circuit in a response conflict task: a PET study. *Brain* 2002;**125**:1995–2004.

37. Alegret M, Junque C, Valldeoriola F, et al. Effects of bilateral subthalamic stimulation on cognitive function in Parkinson disease. *Arch Neurol* 2001;**58**:1223–7.

38. Saint-Cyr JA, Trepanier LL, Kumar R, Lozano AM, Lang AE. Neuropsychological consequences of chronic bilateral stimulation of the subthalamic nucleus in Parkinson's disease. *Brain* 2000;**123** (10):2091–108.

39. Morrison CE, Borod JC, Perrine K, et al. Neuropsychological functioning following bilateral subthalamic nucleus stimulation in Parkinson's disease. *Arch Clin Neuropsychol* 2004;**19**:165–81.

40. Gironell A, Kulisevsky J, Rami L, et al. Effects of pallidotomy and bilateral subthalamic stimulation on cognitive function in Parkinson disease. A controlled comparative study. *J Neurol* 2003;**250**:917–23.

41. De Gaspari D, Siri C, Di Gioia M, et al. Clinical correlates and cognitive underpinnings of verbal fluency impairment after chronic subthalamic stimulation in Parkinson's disease. *Parkinsonism Relat Disord* 2006;**12**:289–95.

42. De Gaspari D, Siri C, Landi A, et al. Clinical and neuropsychological follow up at 12 months in patients with complicated Parkinson's disease treated with subcutaneous apomorphine infusion or deep brain stimulation of the subthalamic nucleus. *J Neurol Neurosurg Psychiatry* 2006;**77**:450–3.

43. Okun MS, Foote KD. A mnemonic for Parkinson disease patients considering DBS: a tool to improve perceived outcome of surgery. *Neurologist* 2004;**10**:290.

44. Okun MS, Rodriguez RL, Foote KD, et al. A case-based review of troubleshooting deep brain stimulator issues in movement and neuropsychiatric disorders. *Parkinsonism Relat Disord* 2008;**14**:532–8.

45. Seijo FJ, Alvarez-Vega MA, Gutierrez JC, Fdez-Glez F, Lozano B. Complications in subthalamic nucleus stimulation surgery for treatment of Parkinson's disease. Review of 272 procedures. *Acta neurochir* 2007;**149**:867–75; discussion 876.

46. Hariz MI. Complications of deep brain stimulation surgery. *Mov Disord* 2002;**17**:S162–6.

47. Beric A, Kelly PJ, Rezai A, et al. Complications of deep brain stimulation surgery. *Stereotact Funct Neurosurg* 2001;**77**:73–8.

48. Oh MY, Abosch A, Kim SH, Lang AE, Lozano AM. Long-term hardware-related complications of deep brain stimulation. *Neurosurgery* 2002;**50**:1268–74; discussion 1274–6.

49. Hariz MI, Fodstad H. Do microelectrode techniques increase accuracy or decrease risks in pallidotomy and deep brain stimulation? A critical review of the literature. *Stereotact Funct Neurosurg* 1999;**72**:157–69.

50. Palur RS, Berk C, Schulzer M, Honey CR. A metaanalysis comparing the results of pallidotomy performed using microelectrode recording or macroelectrode stimulation. *J Neurosurg* 2002;**96**:1058–62.

51. Gorgulho A, De Salles AA, Frighetto L, Behnke E. Incidence of hemorrhage associated with electrophysiological studies performed using macroelectrodes and microelectrodes in functional neurosurgery. *J Neurosurg* 2005;**102**:888–96.

52. Umemura A, Jaggi JL, Hurtig HI, et al. Deep brain stimulation for movement disorders: morbidity and mortality in 109 patients. *J Neurosurg* 2003;**98**:779–84.

53. Binder DK, Rau GM, Starr PA. Risk factors for hemorrhage during microelectrode-guided deep brain stimulator implantation for movement disorders. *Neurosurgery* 2005;**56**:722–32; discussion 732.

54. Sansur CA, Frysinger RC, Pouratian N, et al. Incidence of symptomatic hemorrhage after stereotactic electrode placement. *J Neurosurg* 2007;**107**:998–1003.

55. Broderick J, Connolly S, Feldmann E, et al. Guidelines for the management of spontaneous intracerebral hemorrhage in adults: 2007 update: a guideline from the American Heart Association/American Stroke Association, Stroke Council, High Blood Pressure Research Council, and the Quality of Care and Outcomes in Research Interdisciplinary Working Group. *Stroke* 2007;**38**:2001–23.

56. van den Bergh WM, van der Schaaf I, van Gijn J. The spectrum of presentations of venous infarction caused by deep cerebral vein thrombosis. *Neurology* 2005;**65**:192–6.

57. Morcos Z. The spectrum of presentations of venous infarction caused by deep cerebral vein thrombosis. *Neurology* 2006;**66**:1284; author reply.

58. Ferro JM, Canhao P. Acute treatment of cerebral venous and dural sinus thrombosis. *Curr Treat Options Neurol* 2008;**10**:126–37.

59. Zeng L, Derex L, Maarrawi J, et al. Lifesaving decompressive craniectomy in 'malignant' cerebral venous infarction. *Eur J Neurol* 2007;**14**:e27–8.

60. Masuhr F, Einhaupl K. Treatment of cerebral venous and sinus thrombosis. *Front Neurol Neurosci* 2008;**23**:132–43.

61. Ferro JM, Canhao P, Bousser MG, Stam J, Barinagarrementeria F. Early seizures in cerebral vein and dural sinus thrombosis: risk factors and role of antiepileptics. *Stroke* 2008;**39**:1152–8.

62. Hamani C, Richter E, Schwalb JM, Lozano AM. Bilateral subthalamic nucleus stimulation for Parkinson's disease: a systematic review of the clinical

literature. *Neurosurgery* 2005;**56**:1313–21; discussion 1321–4.

63. Inci S, Erbengi A, Berker M. Pulmonary embolism in neurosurgical patients. *Surg Neurol* 1995;**43**:123–8; discussion 128–9.

64. Muir KW. The PREVAIL trial and low-molecular-weight heparin for prevention of venous thromboembolism. *Stroke* 2008;**39**:2174–6.

65. Patrono C, Baigent C, Hirsh J, Roth G. Antiplatelet drugs: American College of Chest Physicians Evidence-Based Clinical Practice Guidelines (8th Edition). *Chest* 2008;**133**:199S–233S.

66. Lee AY, Levine MN, Baker RI, et al. Low-molecular-weight heparin versus a coumarin for the prevention of recurrent venous thromboembolism in patients with cancer. *N Engl J Med* 2003;**349**:146–53.

67. Voges J, Hilker R, Botzel K, et al. Thirty days complication rate following surgery performed for deep-brain-stimulation. *Mov Disord* 2007;**22**:1486–9.

68. Marik PE. Aspiration pneumonitis and aspiration pneumonia. *N Engl J Med* 2001;**344**:665–71.

69. Deep-Brain Stimulation for Parkinson's Disease Study Group. Deep-brain stimulation of the subthalamic nucleus or the pars interna of the globus pallidus in Parkinson's disease. *N Engl J Med* 2001;**345**:956–63.

70. Volkmann J, Allert N, Voges J, et al. Safety and efficacy of pallidal or subthalamic nucleus stimulation in advanced PD. *Neurology* 2001;**56**:548–51.

71. Okun MS, Tagliati M, Pourfar M, et al. Management of referred deep brain stimulation failures: a retrospective analysis from two movement disorders centers. *Arch Neurol* 2005;**62**:1250–5.

72. Lyons KE, Wilkinson SB, Overman J, Pahwa R. Surgical and hardware complications of subthalamic stimulation: a series of 160 procedures. *Neurology* 2004;**63**:612–16.

73. Benabid AL, Koudsie A, Benazzouz A, Le Bas JF, Pollak P. Imaging of subthalamic nucleus and ventralis intermedius of the thalamus. *Mov Disord* 2002;**17** (Suppl 3):S123–9.

74. Sillay KA, Larson PS, Starr PA. Deep brain stimulator hardware-related infections: incidence and management in a large series. *Neurosurgery* 2008;**62**:360–6; discussion 366–7.

75. Levy RM, Lamb S, Adams JE. Treatment of chronic pain by deep brain stimulation: long term follow-up and review of the literature. *Neurosurgery* 1987;**21**:885–93.

76. Seal LA, Paul-Cheadle D. A systems approach to preoperative surgical patient skin preparation. *Am J Infect Control* 2004;**32**:57–62.

77. Miyagi Y, Shima F, Ishido K. Implantation of deep brain stimulation electrodes in unshaved patients. Technical note. *J Neurosurg* 2002;**97**:1476–8.

78. Masterson TM, Rodeheaver GT, Morgan RF, Edlich RF. Bacteriologic evaluation of electric clippers for surgical hair removal. *Am J Surg* 1984;**148**:301–2.

79. Medtronic. *Deep Brain Stimulation 3387/89 Lead Kit: Implant Manual.* Minneapolis: Medtronic, Inc.; 2000.

80. Sherif C, Dorfer C, Kalteis K, et al. Deep brain pulse-generator and lead-extensions: subjective sensations related to measured parameters. *Mov Disord* 2008;**23**:1036–40.

81. Hariz MI, Johansson F. Hardware failure in parkinsonian patients with chronic subthalamic nucleus stimulation is a medical emergency. *Mov Disord* 2001;**16**:166–8.

82. Schwalb JM, Riina HA, Skolnick B, et al. Revision of deep brain stimulator for tremor. Technical note. *J Neurosurg* 2001;**94**:1010–12.

83. Blomstedt P, Hariz MI. Hardware-related complications of deep brain stimulation: a ten year experience. *Acta Neurochir* 2005;**147**:1061–4; discussion 1064.

84. Machado AG, Hiremath GK, Salazar F, Rezai AR. Fracture of subthalamic nucleus deep brain stimulation hardware as a result of compulsive manipulation: case report. *Neurosurgery* 2005;**57**: E1318.

85. Cardoso AF, Almeida GM. Twiddler syndrome. *Arq Bras Cardiol* 2008;**90**:E15.

86. Dursun I, Yesildag O, Soylu K, et al. Late pacemaker twiddler syndrome. *Clin Res Cardiol* 2006;**95**:547–9.

87. Fahraeus T, Hoijer CJ. Early pacemaker twiddler syndrome. *Europace* 2003;**5**:279–81.

88. Geissinger G, Neal JH. Spontaneous twiddler's syndrome in a patient with a deep brain stimulator. *Surg Neurol* 2007;**68**:454–6; discussion 456.

89. Farris S, Vitek J, Giroux ML. Deep brain stimulation hardware complications: The role of electrode impedance and current measurements. *Mov Disord* 2008 **23**:755–60.

90. Benezet-Mazuecos J, Benezet J, Ortega-Carnicer J. Pacemaker twiddler syndrome. *Eur Heart J* 2007;**28**:2000.

91. Yianni J, Nandi D, Shad A, et al. Increased risk of lead fracture and migration in dystonia compared with other movement disorders following deep brain stimulation. *J Clin Neurosci* 2004;**11**:243–5.

92. Favre J, Taha JM, Steel T, Burchiel KJ. Anchoring of deep brain stimulation electrodes using a microplate. Technical note. *J Neurosurg* 1996;**85**:1181–3.

93. Alesch F, Pinter MM, Helscher RJ, et al. Stimulation of the ventral intermediate thalamic nucleus in tremor dominated Parkinson's disease and essential tremor. *Acta Neurochir* 1995;**136**:75–81.

94. Kiss ZH, Anderson T, Hansen T, et al. Neural substrates of microstimulation-evoked tingling: a chronaxie study in human somatosensory thalamus. *Eur J Neurosci* 2003;**18**:728–32.

95. Deuschl G, Herzog J, Kleiner-Fisman G, et al. Deep brain stimulation: postoperative issues. *Mov Disord* 2006;**21**:S219–37.

96. Ashby P, Kim YJ, Kumar R, Lang AE, Lozano AM. Neurophysiological effects of stimulation through electrodes in the human subthalamic nucleus. *Brain* 1999;**122**(Pt 10):1919–31.

97. Krack P, Fraix V, Mendes A, Benabid AL, Pollak P. Postoperative management of subthalamic nucleus stimulation for Parkinson's disease. *Mov Disord* 2002;**17**:S188–97.

98. Albanese A, Nordera GP, Caraceni T, Moro E. Long-term ventralis intermedius thalamic stimulation for parkinsonian tremor. Italian Registry for Neuromodulation in Movement Disorders. *Adv Neurol* 1999;**80**:631–4.

99. Kumar K, Kelly M, Toth C. Deep brain stimulation of the ventral intermediate nucleus of the thalamus for control of tremors in Parkinson's disease and essential tremor. *Stereotact Funct Neurosurg* 1999;**72**:47–61.

100. Limousin P, Speelman JD, Gielen F, Janssens M. Multicentre European study of thalamic stimulation in parkinsonian and essential tremor. *J Neurol Neurosurg Psychiatry* 1999;**66**:289–96.

101. Tamma F, Caputo E, Chiesa V, et al. Anatomo-clinical correlation of intraoperative stimulation-induced side-effects during HF-DBS of the subthalamic nucleus. *Neurol Sci* 2002;**23**(Suppl 2):S109–10.

102. Benabid AL, Pollak P, Gao D, et al. Chronic electrical stimulation of the ventralis intermedius nucleus of the thalamus as a treatment of movement disorders. *J Neurosurg* 1996;**84**:203–14.

103. Limousin-Dowsey P, Pollak P, Van Blercom N, et al. Thalamic, subthalamic nucleus and internal pallidum stimulation in Parkinson's disease. *J Neurol* 1999;**246**(Suppl 2):II42–5.

104. Kumar K, Kelly M, Toth C. Deep brain stimulation of the ventral intermediate nucleus of the thalamus for control of tremors in Parkinson's disease and essential tremor. *Stereotact Funct Neurosurg* 1999;**72**:47–61.

105. Tavella A, Bergamasco B, Bosticco E, et al. Deep brain stimulation of the subthalamic nucleus in Parkinson's disease: long-term follow-up. *Neurol Sci* 2002;**23** (Suppl 2):S111–12.

106. Kleiner-Fisman G, Fisman DN, Sime E, et al. Long-term follow up of bilateral deep brain stimulation of the subthalamic nucleus in patients with advanced Parkinson disease. *J Neurosurg* 2003;**99**:489–95.

107. Valldeoriola F, Pilleri M, Tolosa E, et al. Bilateral subthalamic stimulation monotherapy in advanced Parkinson's disease: long-term follow-up of patients. *Mov Disord* 2002;**17**:125–32.

108. Pinto S, Gentil M, Krack P, et al. Changes induced by levodopa and subthalamic nucleus stimulation on parkinsonian speech. *Mov Disord* 2005;**20**:1507–15.

109. Ramig LO, Sapir S, Countryman S, et al. Intensive voice treatment (LSVT) for patients with Parkinson's disease: a 2 year follow up. *J Neurol Neurosurg Psychiatry* 2001;**71**:493–8.

110. Ramig LO, Sapir S, Fox C, Countryman S. Changes in vocal loudness following intensive voice treatment (LSVT) in individuals with Parkinson's disease: a comparison with untreated patients and normal age-matched controls. *Mov Disord* 2001;**16**:79–83.

111. Sapir S, Ramig LO, Hoyt P, et al. Speech loudness and quality 12 months after intensive voice treatment (LSVT) for Parkinson's disease: a comparison with an alternative speech treatment. *Folia Phoniatr Logop* 2002;**54**:296–303.

112. Bejjani BP, Gervais D, Arnulf I, et al. Axial parkinsonian symptoms can be improved: the role of levodopa and bilateral subthalamic stimulation. *J Neurol Neurosurg Psychiatry* 2000;**68**:595–600.

113. Pahwa R, Lyons KL, Wilkinson SB, et al. Bilateral thalamic stimulation for the treatment of essential tremor. *Neurology* 1999;**53**:1447–50.

114. Felice KJ, Keilson GR, Schwartz WJ. 'Rubral' gait ataxia. *Neurology* 1990;**40**:1004–5.

115. Limousin P, Krack P, Pollak P, et al. Electrical stimulation of the subthalamic nucleus in advanced Parkinson's disease. *N Engl J Med* 1998;**339**:1105–11.

116. Forget R, Tozlovanu V, Iancu A, Boghen D. Botulinum toxin improves lid opening delays in blepharospasm-associated apraxia of lid opening. *Neurology* 2002;**58**:1843–6.

117. Voon V, Kubu C, Krack P, Houeto JL, Troster AI. Deep brain stimulation: neuropsychological and neuropsychiatric issues. *Mov Disord* 2006;**21**(Suppl 14): S305–27.

118. Hariz MI, Johansson F, Shamsgovara P, et al. Bilateral subthalamic nucleus stimulation in a parkinsonian

patient with preoperative deficits in speech and cognition: persistent improvement in mobility but increased dependency: a case study. *Mov Disord* 2000;**15**:136–9.

119. Houeto JL, Mesnage V, Mallet L, et al. Behavioural disorders, Parkinson's disease and subthalamic stimulation. *J Neurol Neurosurg Psychiatry* 2002;**72**:701–7.

120. Molinuevo JL, Valldeoriola F, Tolosa E, et al. Levodopa withdrawal after bilateral subthalamic nucleus stimulation in advanced Parkinson disease. *Arch Neurol* 2000;**57**:983–8.

121. Herzog J, Volkmann J, Krack P, et al. Two-year follow-up of subthalamic deep brain stimulation in Parkinson's disease. *Mov Disord* 2003;**18**: 1332–7.

122. Ostergaard K, Sunde N, Dupont E. Effects of bilateral stimulation of the subthalamic nucleus in patients with severe Parkinson's disease and motor fluctuations. *Mov Disord* 2002;**17**:693–700.

123. Rodriguez-Oroz MC, Obeso JA, Lang AE, et al. Bilateral deep brain stimulation in Parkinson's disease: a multicentre study with 4 years follow-up. *Brain* 2005;**128**:2240–9.

124. Doshi PK, Chhaya N, Bhatt MH. Depression leading to attempted suicide after bilateral subthalamic nucleus stimulation for Parkinson's disease. *Mov Disord* 2002;**17**:1084–5.

125. Voon V, Moro E, Saint-Cyr JA, Lozano AM, Lang AE. Psychiatric symptoms following surgery for Parkinson's disease with an emphasis on subthalamic stimulation. *Adv Neurol* 2005;**96**:130–47.

126. Albin RL, Young AB, Penney JB. The functional anatomy of basal ganglia disorders. *Trends Neurosci* 1989;**12**:366–75.

127. Pazo JH, Belforte JE. Basal ganglia and functions of the autonomic nervous system. *Cell Mol Neurobiol* 2002;**22**:645–54.

128. Sauleau P, Raoul S, Lallement F, et al. Motor and non motor effects during intraoperative subthalamic stimulation for Parkinson's disease. *J Neurol* 2005;**252**:457–64.

129. Holmberg B, Corneliusson O, Elam M. Bilateral stimulation of nucleus subthalamicus in advanced Parkinson's disease: no effects on, and of, autonomic dysfunction. *Mov Disord* 2005;**20**:976–81.

130. Kaufmann H, Bhattacharya KF, Voustianiouk A, Gracies JM. Stimulation of the subthalamic nucleus increases heart rate in patients with Parkinson disease. *Neurology* 2002;**59**:1657–8.

131. Thobois S, Mertens P, Guenot M, et al. Subthalamic nucleus stimulation in Parkinson's disease:

132. Esselink RA, de Bie RM, de Haan RJ, et al. Unilateral pallidotomy versus bilateral subthalamic nucleus stimulation in PD: a randomized trial. *Neurology* 2004;**62**:201–7.

133. Krause M, Fogel W, Heck A, et al. Deep brain stimulation for the treatment of Parkinson's disease: subthalamic nucleus versus globus pallidus internus. *J Neurol Neurosurg Psychiatry* 2001;**70**:464–70.

134. Voon V, Hassan K, Zurowski M, et al. Prevalence of repetitive and reward-seeking behaviors in Parkinson disease. *Neurology* 2006;**67**:1254–7.

135. Romito LM, Scerrati M, Contarino MF, et al. Long-term follow up of subthalamic nucleus stimulation in Parkinson's disease. *Neurology* 2002;**58**:1546–50.

136. Castelli L, Perozzo P, Genesia ML, et al. Sexual well being in parkinsonian patients after deep brain stimulation of the subthalamic nucleus. *J Neurol Neurosurg Psychiatry* 2004;**75**:1260–4.

137. Romito LM, Raja M, Daniele A, et al. Transient mania with hypersexuality after surgery for high frequency stimulation of the subthalamic nucleus in Parkinson's disease. *Mov Disord* 2002;**17**:1371–4.

138. Jimenez-Jimenez FJ, Sayed Y, Garcia-Soldevilla MA, Barcenilla B. Possible zoophilia associated with dopaminergic therapy in Parkinson disease. *Ann Pharmacother* 2002;**36**:1178–9.

139. Klos KJ, Bower JH, Josephs KA, Matsumoto JY, Ahlskog JE. Pathological hypersexuality predominantly linked to adjuvant dopamine agonist therapy in Parkinson's disease and multiple system atrophy. *Parkinsonism Relat Disord* 2005;**11**:381–6.

140. Ivanco LS, Bohnen NI. Effects of donepezil on compulsive hypersexual behavior in Parkinson disease: a single case study. *Am J Ther* 2005;**12**:467–8.

141. Gironell A, Kulisevsky J, Rami L, et al. Effects of pallidotomy and bilateral subthalamic stimulation on cognitive function in Parkinson disease. A controlled comparative study. *J Neurol* 2003;**250**:917–23.

142. Barichella M, Marczewska AM, Mariani C, et al. Body weight gain rate in patients with Parkinson's disease and deep brain stimulation. *Mov Disord* 2003;**18**:1337–40.

143. Macia F, Perlemoine C, Coman I, et al. Parkinson's disease patients with bilateral subthalamic deep brain stimulation gain weight. *Mov Disord* 2004;**19**:206–12.

144. Montaurier C, Morio B, Bannier S, et al. Mechanisms of body weight gain in patients with Parkinson's disease after subthalamic stimulation. *Brain* 2007;**130**:1808–18.

clinical evaluation of 18 patients. *J Neurol* 2002;**249**:529–34.

145. Kumar R, Lang AE, Rodriguez-Oroz MC, et al. Deep brain stimulation of the globus pallidus pars interna in advanced Parkinson's disease. *Neurology* 2000; **55**:S34–9.

146. Kirschman DL, Milligan B, Wilkinson S, et al. Pallidotomy microelectrode targeting: neurophysiology-based target refinement. *Neurosurgery* 2000;**46**:613–22; discussion 622–4.

147. Biousse V, Newman NJ, Carroll C, et al. Visual fields in patients with posterior GPi pallidotomy. *Neurology* 1998;**50**:258–65.

148. Lang AE, Houeto JL, Krack P, et al. Deep brain stimulation: preoperative issues. *Mov Disord* 2006;**21**: S171–96.

149. Moro E, Lang AE. Criteria for deep-brain stimulation in Parkinson's disease: review and analysis. *Expert Rev Neurother* 2006;**6**:1695–705.

150. Hughes AJ, Daniel SE, Ben-Shlomo Y, Lees AJ. The accuracy of diagnosis of parkinsonian syndromes in a specialist movement disorder service. *Brain* 2002;**125**:861–70.

151. Charles PD, Van Blercom N, Krack P, et al. Predictors of effective bilateral subthalamic nucleus stimulation for PD. *Neurology* 2002;**59**:932–4.

152. Okun MS, Fernandez HH, Pedraza O, et al. Development and initial validation of a screening tool for Parkinson disease surgical candidates. *Neurology* 2004;**63**:161–3.

153. Marjama-Lyons J, Okun MS. *Parkinson Disease: Guide to Deep Brain Stimulation*. Miami, FL: National Parkinson Foundation; 2007.

154. Kronenbuerger M, Fromm C, Block F, et al. On-demand deep brain stimulation for essential tremor: a report on four cases. *Mov Disord* 2006;**21**:401–5.

155. Devlin N, Williams A. Valuing quality of life: results for New Zealand health professionals. *N Z Med J* 1999;**112**:68–71.

156. Wiklund I. The Nottingham Health Profile–a measure of health-related quality of life. *Scand J Prim Health Care Suppl* 1990;**1**:15–18.

157. Hobson P, Holden A, Meara J. Measuring the impact of Parkinson's disease with the Parkinson's Disease Quality of Life questionnaire. *Age Ageing* 1999;**28**:341–6.

158. Jenkinson C, Fitzpatrick R, Argyle M. The Nottingham Health Profile: an analysis of its sensitivity in differentiating illness groups. *Soc Sci Med* 1988;**27**:1411–14.

159. Sullivan M, Karlsson J, Ware JE, Jr. The Swedish SF-36 Health Survey–I. Evaluation of data quality, scaling assumptions, reliability and construct validity across general populations in Sweden. *Soc Sci Med* 1995;**41**:1349–58.

160. Hunt SM, McKenna SP. Validating the SF-36. *BMJ* 1992; **305**:645; author reply 646.

161. Hagell P, Whalley D, McKenna SP, Lindvall O. Health status measurement in Parkinson's disease: validity of the PDQ-39 and Nottingham Health Profile. *Mov Disord* 2003;**18**:773–83.

162. Thorsen H, McKenna S, Tennant A, Holstein P. Nottingham health profile scores predict the outcome and support aggressive revascularisation for critical ischaemia. *Eur J Vasc Endovasc Surg* 2002;**23**:495–9.

163. Den Oudsten BL, Van Heck GL, De Vries J. The suitability of patient-based measures in the field of Parkinson's disease: a systematic review. *Mov Disord* 2007;**22**:1390–401.

164. Damiano AM, Snyder C, Strausser B, Willian MK. A review of health-related quality-of-life concepts and measures for Parkinson's disease. *Qual Life Res* 1999;**8**:235–43.

165. Schulzer M, Mak E, Calne SM. The psychometric properties of the Parkinson's Impact Scale (PIMS) as a measure of quality of life in Parkinson's disease. *Parkinsonism Relat Disord* 2003;**9**:291–4.

166. Diamond A, Jankovic J. The effect of deep brain stimulation on quality of life in movement disorders. *J Neurol Neurosurg Psychiatry* 2005;**76**:1188–93.

167. Calne SM, Mak E, Hall J, et al. Validating a quality-of-life scale in caregivers of patients with Parkinson's disease: Parkinson's Impact Scale (PIMS). *Adv Neurol* 2003;**91**:115–22.

168. Jenkinson C, Fitzpatrick R, Peto V, Greenhall R, Hyman N. The Parkinson's Disease Questionnaire (PDQ-39): development and validation of a Parkinson's disease summary index score. *Age Ageing* 1997;**26**:353–7.

169. Peto V, Jenkinson C, Fitzpatrick R, Greenhall R. The development and validation of a short measure of functioning and well being for individuals with Parkinson's disease. *Qual Life Res* 1995;**4**:241–8.

170. Folstein MF, Folstein SE, McHugh PR. "Mini-mental state". A practical method for grading the cognitive state of patients for the clinician. *J Psychiatr Res* 1975;**12**:189–98.

171. Gardner R, Jr, Oliver-Munoz S, Fisher L, Empting L. Mattis Dementia Rating Scale: internal reliability study using a diffusely impaired population. *J Clin Neuropsychol* 1981;**3**:271–5.

172. Wechsler D. *Wechsler Adult Intelligence Scale (WAIS-3R)*, 3rd edn. San Antonio, TX: Harcourt Assessment; 1997.

173. Lhermitte F, Pillon B, Serdaru M. Human autonomy and the frontal lobes. Part I: Imitation and utilization behavior: a neuropsychological study of 75 patients. *Ann Neurol* 1986;**19**:326–34.

174. Nelson HE. A modified card sorting test sensitive to frontal lobe defects. *Cortex* 1976;**12**:313–24.

175. Giovagnoli AR, Del Pesce M, Mascheroni S, et al. Trail making test: normative values from 287 normal adult controls. *Ital J Neurol Sci* 1996;**17**:305–9.

176. Miner T, Ferraro FR. The role of speed of processing, inhibitory mechanisms, and presentation order in trail-making test performance. *Brain Cogn* 1998;**38**:246–53.

177. Tombaugh TN, Kozak J, Rees L. Normative data stratified by age and education for two measures of verbal fluency: FAS and animal naming. *Arch Clin Neuropsychol* 1999;**14**:167–77.

178. Benton AL, Hamsher K. *Multilingual Aphasia Examination.* Iowa City, Iowa: AJA Associates; 1989.

179. Arbuthnott K, Frank J. Trail making test, part B as a measure of executive control: validation using a set-switching paradigm. *J Clin Exp Neuropsychol* 2000;**22**:518–28.

180. Amodio P, Wenin H, Del Piccolo F, et al. Variability of trail making test, symbol digit test and line trait test in normal people. A normative study taking into account age-dependent decline and sociobiological variables. *Aging Clin Exp Res* 2002;**14**:117–31.

181. Mascolo MF, Hirtle SC. Verbal coding and the elimination of Stroop interference in a matching task. *Am J Psychol* 1990;**103**:195–215.

182. Van der Elst W, Van Boxtel MP, Van Breukelen GJ, Jolles J. Detecting the significance of changes in performance on the Stroop Color-Word Test, Rey's Verbal Learning Test, and the Letter Digit Substitution Test: the regression-based change approach. *J Int Neuropsychol Soc* 2008;**14**:71–80.

183. Flowers KA, Robertson C. The effect of Parkinson's disease on the ability to maintain a mental set. *J Neurol Neurosurg Psychiatry* 1985;**48**:517–29.

184. Wechsler D. *Wechsler Memory Scale.* San Antonio, TX: The Psychological Corporation; 1997.

185. Owen AM, Beksinska M, James M, et al. Visuospatial memory deficits at different stages of Parkinson's disease. *Neuropsychologia* 1993;**31**:627–44.

186. Cooper JA, Sagar HJ, Jordan N, Harvey NS, Sullivan EV. Cognitive impairment in early, untreated Parkinson's disease and its relationship to motor disability. *Brain* 1991;**114** (Pt 5):2095–122.

187. Wiens AN, Fuller KH, Crossen JR. Paced Auditory Serial Addition Test: adult norms and moderator variables. *J Clin Exp Neuropsychol* 1997;**19**:473–83.

188. Tombaugh TN. A comprehensive review of the Paced Auditory Serial Addition Test (PASAT). *Arch Clin Neuropsychol* 2006;**21**:53–76.

189. Shapiro AM, Benedict RH, Schretlen D, Brandt J. Construct and concurrent validity of the Hopkins Verbal Learning Test-revised. *Clin Neuropsychol* 1999;**13**:348–58.

190. Frank RM, Byrne GJ. The clinical utility of the Hopkins Verbal Learning Test as a screening test for mild dementia. *Int J Geriatr Psychiatry* 2000;**15**:317–24.

191. Ryan JJ, Geisser ME. Validity and diagnostic accuracy of an alternate form of the Rey Auditory Verbal Learning Test. *Arch Clin Neuropsychol* 1986;**1**:209–17.

192. Poreh A. Analysis of mean learning of normal participants on the Rey Auditory-Verbal Learning Test. *Psychol Assess* 2005;**17**:191–9.

193. Pillon B, Deweer B, Agid Y, Dubois B. Explicit memory in Alzheimer's, Huntington's, and Parkinson's diseases. *Arch Neurol* 1993;**50**:374–9.

194. Cockburn J. Performance on the Tower of London test after severe head injury. *J Int Neuropsychol Soc* 1995;**1**:537–44.

195. Delis DC, Kramer JH, Kaplan E, Holdnack J. Reliability and validity of the Delis-Kaplan Executive Function System: an update. *J Int Neuropsychol Soc* 2004;**10**:301–3.

196. Homack S, Lee D, Riccio CA. Test review: Delis-Kaplan executive function system. *J Clin Exp Neuropsychol* 2005;**27**:599–609.

197. Kent PS, Luszcz MA. A review of the Boston Naming Test and multiple-occasion normative data for older adults on 15-item versions. *Clin Neuropsychol* 2002;**16**:555–74.

198. Calero MD, Arnedo ML, Navarro E, Ruiz-Pedrosa M, Carnero C. Usefulness of a 15-item version of the Boston Naming Test in neuropsychological assessment of low-educational elders with dementia. *J Gerontol B Psychol Sci Soc Sci* 2002;**57**:P187–91.

199. Tombaugh TN, Hubley AM. The 60-item Boston Naming Test: norms for cognitively intact adults aged 25 to 88 years. *J Clin Exp Neuropsychol* 1997;**19**:922–32.

200. Gladsjo JA, Schuman CC, Evans JD, et al. Norms for letter and category fluency: demographic corrections for age, education, and ethnicity. *Assessment* 1999;**6**:147–78.

201. Sunderland T, Hill JL, Mellow AM, et al. Clock drawing in Alzheimer's disease. A novel measure of dementia severity. *J Am Geriatr Soc* 1989;**37**:725–9.

202. Janvin C, Aarsland D, Larsen JP, Hugdahl K. Neuropsychological profile of patients with

129

Parkinson's disease without dementia. *Dement Geriatr Cogn Disord* 2003;**15**:126–31.

203. Warrington EK, James M. *The Visual Object and Space Perception Battery.* Bury St Edmunds, Suffolk, UK: Thames Valley Test Company; 1991.

204. Mason CF, Ganzler H. Adult Norms for the Shipley Institute of Living Scale and Hooper Visual Organization Test Based on Age and Education. *J Gerontol* 1964;**19**:419–24.

205. Merten T, Beal C. An analysis of the Hooper Visual Organization Test with neurological patients. *Clin Neuropsychol* 1999;**13**:521–9.

206. Schretlen DJ, Pearlson GD, Anthony JC, Yates KO. Determinants of Benton Facial Recognition Test performance in normal adults. *Neuropsychology* 2001;**15**:405–10.

207. Starkstein SE, Mayberg HS, Preziosi TJ, et al. Reliability, validity, and clinical correlates of apathy in Parkinson's disease. *J Neuropsychiatry Clin Neurosci* 1992;**4**:134–9.

208. Sockeel P, Dujardin K, Devos D, et al. The Lille apathy rating scale (LARS), a new instrument for detecting and quantifying apathy: validation in Parkinson's disease. *J Neurol Neurosurg Psychiatry* 2006;**77**:579–84.

209. Bruss GS, Gruenberg AM, Goldstein RD, Barber JP. Hamilton Anxiety Rating Scale Interview Guide: joint interview and test-retest methods for interrater reliability. *Psychiatry Res* 1994;**53**:191–202.

210. Leentjens AF, Verhey FR, Lousberg R, Spitsbergen H, Wilmink FW. The validity of the Hamilton and Montgomery-Asberg depression rating scales as screening and diagnostic tools for depression in Parkinson's disease. *Int J Geriatr Psychiatry* 2000;**15**:644–9.

211. Weintraub D, Oehlberg KA, Katz IR, Stern MB. Test characteristics of the 15-item geriatric depression scale and Hamilton depression rating scale in Parkinson disease. *Am J Geriatr Psychiatry* 2006;**14**:169–75.

212. Visser M, Leentjens AF, Marinus J, Stiggelbout AM, van Hilten JJ. Reliability and validity of the Beck depression inventory in patients with Parkinson's disease. *Mov Disord* 2006;**21**:668–72.

213. Ertan FS, Ertan T, Kızıltan G, Uygucgil H. Reliability and validity of the Geriatric Depression Scale in depression in Parkinson's disease. *J Neurol Neurosurg Psychiatry* 2005;**76**:1445–7.

214. Thurber S, Snow M, Honts CR. The Zung Self-Rating Depression Scale: convergent validity and diagnostic discrimination. *Assessment* 2002;**9**:401–5.

215. Biggs JT, Wylie LT, Ziegler VE. Validity of the Zung Self-rating Depression Scale. *Br J Psychiatry* 1978;**132**:381–5.

216. Young RC, Biggs JT, Ziegler VE, Meyer DA. A rating scale for mania: reliability, validity and sensitivity. *Br J Psychiatry* 1978;**133**:429–35.

217. Steiner M, Streiner DL. Validation of a revised visual analog scale for premenstrual mood symptoms: results from prospective and retrospective trials. *Can J Psychiatry* 2005;**50**:327–32.

218. Kim SW, Dysken MW, Kuskowski M. The Yale-Brown Obsessive-Compulsive Scale: a reliability and validity study. *Psychiatry Res* 1990;**34**:99–106.

219. Goodman WK, Price LH, Rasmussen SA, et al. The Yale-Brown Obsessive Compulsive Scale. I. Development, use, and reliability. *Arch Gen Psychiatry* 1989;**46**:1006–11.

220. Goodman WK, Price LH, Rasmussen SA, et al. The Yale-Brown Obsessive Compulsive Scale. II. Validity. *Arch Gen Psychiatry* 1989;**46**:1012–16.

221. Cummings JL, Mega M, Gray K, et al. The Neuropsychiatric Inventory: comprehensive assessment of psychopathology in dementia. *Neurology* 2004;**44**:2308–14.

222. Brandstaedter D, Spieker S, Ulm G, et al. Development and evaluation of the Parkinson Psychosis Questionnaire: A screening-instrument for the early diagnosis of drug-induced psychosis in Parkinson's disease. *J Neurol* 2005;**252**:1060–6.

223. Voges J, Volkmann J, Allert N, et al. Bilateral high-frequency stimulation in the subthalamic nucleus for the treatment of Parkinson disease: correlation of therapeutic effect with anatomical electrode position. *J Neurosurg* 2002;**96**:269–79.

Chapter 10

Implementing deep brain stimulation into practice
Models of patient care
Stephen Grill

The goal of a deep brain stimulation (DBS) program is to treat those patients who have appropriate indications for DBS and are in the referral base for the program. A successful DBS program: (1) identifies suitable patients on a regular basis; (2) undertakes an appropriate evaluation protocol; (3) educates patients and their care partners about DBS; (4) performs the DBS surgery; (5) cares for the patient before and after surgery by programming the stimulators and adjusting medications; and (6) does all of this in an economically feasible manner. Doing this requires a team approach that often includes physicians, nurses, mental health professionals, other medical professionals, and the patient and their care partners. Assembling the necessary evaluation and treatment components for a successful program is the topic discussed in this chapter.

Specifically, this chapter considers how a neurologist specializing in movement disorders should assemble a team (Table 10.1) and organize a standard protocol for accomplishing the necessary procedures.

> Although it may seem easiest to organize a DBS team in a university setting, successful programs can be run out of private practice neurology centers with expertise in movement disorders. It is only necessary that all essential components are present and that the medical professionals act cooperatively, adhering to a specific and deliberate protocol.

A program that has excellent neurosurgeons, movement disorder neurologists, nurses, and psychologists working as a team will not thrive unless there are relationships with referring neurologists and internists/family physicians. These relationships and referral patterns develop over time and are based on physician education, good communication, and the demonstration that patients are handled successfully. Although DBS has been approved by the US Food and Drug Administration for Essential Tremor (ET) since 1997, for Parkinson's disease (PD) since 2002, and for dystonia (under a Humanitarian Device Exemption) since 2003, many physicians are still not familiar with the selection criteria and outcomes for this treatment. Face-to-face educational opportunities with referring neurologists and internists, including lectures and discussions, are helpful in cultivating these relationships. Communication with these physicians at each stage of the evaluation and treatment phases of the DBS protocol is good medicine.

The DBS evaluation protocol is more complex for PD compared to ET and dystonia, so most of the discussion here is focused on PD. Additional specific comments regarding ET and dystonia are presented where appropriate.

The DBS team

> A successful DBS team should operate like a well-oiled machine. Each member of the team should understand their role and communicate their findings in a reliable manner. A monthly multidisciplinary review of upcoming DBS candidates and current patients who may be potential candidates for treatment with DBS should be routinely conducted.

Detailed descriptions of the procedures for patient selection and care are provided in previous chapters. The general roles of the team members are discussed here.

Deep Brain Stimulation Management, ed. William J. Marks, Jr. Published by Cambridge University Press.

Table 10.1 Roles of deep brain stimulation (DBS) personnel

Movement disorder neurologist

Initial screening evaluation of the referred patient

Coordination of other team members

Education of the patient and their care providers

Performance of off-medication and on-medication motor evaluations

Programming of DBS system

Education of referring neurologists and primary care physicians

Neurosurgeon

Neurosurgical evaluation

Education of patient and their care providers

Performance of DBS surgery

Perioperative care of patient

Education of referring neurologists and primary care physicians

Psychologist

Psychological testing

Neurocognitive testing

Psychological treatment, as needed

Referring neurologist

Referral of patient

Communication of history of prior treatment and outcomes

Continued clinical care of patient

Primary care physicians

Medical clearance for surgery

Continued clinical care of patient

Psychiatrist

Psychiatric evaluation and treatment, as needed

Physical, occupational, and speech therapists

Evaluation and treatment, as needed

Movement disorder neurologist

It is the movement disorder neurologist whose task it is to decide if the patient satisfies the clinical criteria that predict a favorable benefit/risk assessment and likelihood of a good outcome with DBS treatment.

The movement disorder neurologist is best able to ensure that a patient indeed has idiopathic PD (or ET or dystonia), rather than another condition,[1] and that the pharmacological management has been optimized before proceeding to DBS surgery. In addition, the movement disorder neurologist must establish that the patient has symptoms that are likely to be helped by DBS, and that they do not have significant contraindications to surgery. Additional responsibilities include coordinating the other team members, education of the patient and care partners, programming (or supervising the programming) of the stimulators, and medication management postoperatively.

Neurosurgeon

The neurosurgeon is responsible for determining that the patient is a DBS surgical candidate and is able to tolerate the surgery. In addition, the neurosurgeon should educate the patient concerning the surgery and must ensure that the patient and family understand the potential risks and expected benefits of the surgery in order for the patient to provide informed consent. Finally, the neurosurgeon must care for the patient in the perioperative period and must communicate operative findings (see Chapter 3) during the surgery to the patient and their family, and to the neurologist responsible for programming the stimulators.

Nurse, nurse practitioner, or physician assistant

Nurses, often advanced practice nurses (such as clinical nurse specialists or nurse practitioners), are commonly members of the DBS team. In many DBS centers, they assist in the preoperative evaluation, perform pre- and post-DBS education for the patient and their care providers, assist in the operating room during DBS surgery, perform DBS programming, and play a vital role in the long-term management of patients. Physician assistants may perform similar roles at some DBS centers.

Psychologist/neuropsychologist

A psychologist provides psychological monitoring and mental healthcare to patients. The neuropsychologist, an individual with specialized training in brain–behavior relationships, is responsible for the performance and interpretation of neurocognitive testing (see Chapter 2). The outcome of the psychological testing is communicated to the movement disorder neurologist. If significant psychiatric illness (especially depression or anxiety) is found, referral to appropriate psychiatrists and psychologists is done; when appropriate, the neurocognitive testing is repeated if and when the psychiatric illness is thought to be well treated. If cognitive dysfunction is found that was not anticipated by the movement disorder neurologist during the initial evaluation, this is communicated to the neurologist and internist and attention is given to finding reversible causes by medication review, evaluation of sleep, etc.

Referring neurologist

Most often, a patient is referred from a neurologist who has cared for the patient for several years, when that neurologist thinks the patient might be helped by DBS. The medical records from this neurologist are valuable information to help understand the effects of prior medication trial/changes, since patient recollection of details of therapy may be poor. It is important to communicate with this physician about the DBS evaluation, and this often involves a telephone conversation to clarify the patient's response to medications. Ordinarily the patient will continue to see the referring neurologist, especially when the patient lives outside the local area of the DBS center. In addition to being good for patient care, the success of a program depends on referrals from other neurologists and therefore good working relationships are important.

Internist/family physician

The patient's primary care physician is an integral member of the team. That physician may have the longest relationship with the patient and may be best able to advise on the patient's co-morbid medical conditions. The role of the internist/family physician is to help with medical clearance for the surgery and ensure that any co-morbid medical conditions are optimally treated. Often if a patient has other significant illnesses, additional specialists (such as cardiologists, endocrinologists, pulmonologists, psychiatrists) will also be involved in the evaluation process. In more rural areas where there may be a paucity of neurologists, internists may be the ones managing movement disorder patients and may thus make the referrals directly to the movement disorder neurologist or DBS center.

Psychiatrist

Though some centers routinely have a psychiatrist who is a member of the team see each patient being considered for DBS,[2] this is not routinely done in all centers.[3,4] This practice may change if studies suggest there is additional benefit of a psychiatric evaluation above and beyond the psychological testing commonly employed. Typically, an in-depth clinical interview is part of the neuropsychological evaluation, and detection of psychiatric concerns is therefore likely to occur as part of this evaluation. If a patient has significant psychiatric illness (for example, depression or anxiety), the patient is referred to both a psychologist for counseling and the psychiatrist for their evaluation and pharmacological treatment.

Physical, occupational, and speech therapists

These therapists play an integral role in the treatment of patients with PD,[5–7] as well as in the treatment of patients with ET and dystonia. Some centers routinely have all patients seen by each of these therapists as part of the DBS evaluation rather than on an as-needed basis. The movement disorder neurologist should make a decision for individual patients whether to refer for therapy evaluations. Often patients are seen in consideration of DBS because of symptoms for which DBS is not indicated or helpful (gait freezing/falls, speech impairment). If these are the main difficulties for the patient, they are counseled that these problems are not reasons to be treated with DBS and they are instead referred to physical or speech therapists.

DBS evaluation protocol

The details of the patient selection process are discussed in Chapter 2. A typical evaluation protocol is presented here in order to illustrate the logistics of carrying out the procedures in an efficient manner. Several additional procedures are often done for academic interest and research purposes, but when not necessary for successful clinical outcome, those are not included here.

There is often a high degree of anxiety concerning the procedure by patients and their families, but many patients are also quite anxious to have the procedure done as soon as possible. It is not unusual for patients to ask if the surgery can be done in a few weeks.

This rush to perform the DBS surgery should be avoided and instead a methodical and consistent approach undertaken. The necessary timeline for evaluation should be explained to the patient at the first encounter. It should be clear to them that the decision to proceed with the surgery requires extensive medical, psychological, and neurological evaluation involving a team of medical professionals, as well as appropriate education of the patient and family about the procedure and realistic expectations about what DBS can and cannot do to treat the patient's symptoms.

Patients who are to proceed with the full DBS evaluation protocol are given a schedule of the evaluations. These include: (1) neurosurgical evaluation; (2) psychological evaluation; (3) medical evaluation; (4) off- and on-medication evaluation (for PD patients). While these are largely separate evaluations, some may occur sequentially or concurrently. Most often the patient has the psychological evaluation and neurological evaluation in the off- and on-medication conditions before seeing the neurosurgeon. Especially for patients traveling long distances to the center, some effort may be made to efficiently coordinate the evaluations to reduce the number of trips the patient has to make. For example, in our center the neurological evaluation and psychological evaluation are often performed at a single visit. It is helpful to give patients written instructions on each of the procedures that must be done.

Initial screening evaluation by movement disorder neurologist

Clinical procedures

Patients being considered for DBS will ordinarily be referred to the movement disorder neurologist by another neurologist who had been managing the patient, or from the clinic/practice of the movement disorder neurologist, because of difficult to control parkinsonian motor fluctuation, tremor, or refractory dystonia. The movement disorder neurologist is to perform a comprehensive initial screening evaluation to determine whether the patient will likely benefit from DBS and therefore whether to proceed with the full DBS evaluation protocol (see Chapter 2).

The consultation report is sent to all of the medical team members, including the neurosurgeon, psychologist, primary care physician, and any other treating physicians/psychologists.

It is common for patients to assume that all aspects of their disease will improve after DBS. Patients must be educated on the expected benefits from DBS and on those symptoms not expected to respond to DBS so that they have appropriate expectations. Patients with dystonia must understand that benefits from DBS may take several months to materialize.

Education

It is helpful to have family or other interested parties present for this discussion and to give the patient literature on the subject, some of which is supplied by support group organizations as well as the manufacturer of the DBS devices.

Because the DBS evaluation protocol, DBS surgery, and postoperative care are complex and sometimes confusing to patients, it is helpful at the initial screening procedure to give a written description of the sequence of events and what to expect at each visit and then to schedule the patient to attend an informational session. We hold such informational sessions on a monthly basis (see below). The opportunity to talk with another patient who has had DBS gives valuable information from a patient perspective, and this can be arranged after this first screening visit.

Educational session for patients and care partners

We have found it helpful to have patients and care partners attend an informational session where the surgical procedure, pre- and postoperative care, and appropriate expectations are discussed in a relaxed, unhurried atmosphere.

Patients should be told in advance that there will be other patients attending, in case they would refrain from attending because of privacy issues. The patient is encouraged to bring whoever ordinarily helps in making important medical decisions with them. A short presentation should cover the indications for the procedure, the evaluation process, what to expect during the surgery, their care after the surgery, and what restrictions they will face after the surgery (such as avoidance of diathermy, strong magnetic fields, MRI except under special circumstances, etc.). Having a demonstration DBS system available, so that the patients can see and hold the hardware, is useful. Patients are given sufficient time to have their questions answered. We hold these sessions on a monthly basis for any patients being considered for DBS to treat PD, ET, and dystonia. The importance of this education cannot be underestimated.

Off- and on-medication evaluation for PD patients
Clinical procedures

> The goal for this evaluation is to assess the severity of motor symptoms in the patient's "off" state, to determine the responsiveness of the patient to dopaminergic medication, and to evaluate the extent of dyskinesia.

The patient comes to the clinic in the "off" state, having not taken medications since midnight the night before (see Chapter 2). To facilitate this for people coming from a distance, a list of nearby hotels should be given to patients so they may stay locally the night before. Although not preferred, if the patient is unable to refrain from taking medication in order to travel to the clinic, the "on" evaluation can be done first and then the "off" evaluation can wait a few hours until the medication has worn off. The timing is flexible, but it may be convenient to see the patient before beginning with routine patients. After an initial examination, including the vital signs, the Unified Parkinson's Disease Rating Scale (UPDRS) (and in our center, timed motor tests) is performed. The patient then takes their medication and is again re-evaluated about an hour later, when their medication is effective. Vital signs and the UPDRS motor scale are repeated, and dyskinesia may be evaluated using standard scales. We routinely record video of patients in both the "off" and "on" states. Once the patient is in their "on" state and feeling well, they ordinarily undergo psychological testing in an effort to efficiently combine visits, but this may be done on another date.

Education

Time is allocated during the day to present to the patient the results of the evaluation (and the

psychological evaluation if already done) and to answer any questions. Also at this visit, written instructions are again provided to the patient about what to expect after the surgery. This includes information about the initial DBS programming session.

Neuropsychological evaluation

> Patients with significant cognitive or psychiatric issues (dementia, psychosis, active depression, and anxiety) are excluded from surgery. Therefore, patients undergo psychological and neurocognitive testing to evaluate for those disorders (see Chapter 2).

In our center, the psychological/neurocognitive evaluation is ordinarily done on the same day as the motor evaluation in order to reduce the number of trips the patient must make to the center. This is helpful for patients traveling a long distance. It also gives the movement disorder neurologist a chance to directly discuss with the psychologist any concerns that arose during the psychological evaluation.

Patients with severe depression are referred for psychiatric and psychological care, and if there is resolution of the depressive symptoms, they may be considered again for DBS surgery.

Neurosurgical evaluation
Clinical procedures

> All patients are seen by the neurosurgeon as part of the comprehensive evaluation to determine the patient's suitability for surgery. This is also a time for the surgeon to discuss the surgical procedure, including the potential risks and complications.

An MRI of the brain is scheduled, since some patients may be excluded from DBS surgery based on the presence of significant abnormality (for example, prior basal ganglia strokes, significant atrophy) on the MRI. Since the patient is typically awake for most of the DBS surgery and the surgeon is dependent on cooperation from the patient during the surgery, this is also a time for the patient and surgeon to develop a cooperative relationship. Although the neurosurgeon is most involved with the patient in the perioperative time period surrounding the initial DBS surgery, there is also a long-standing relationship that develops because of the necessity for replacement of

135

the neurostimulator at regular time intervals, depending on the battery longevity.

Education

> The neurosurgeon should spend time discussing what to expect during the surgery and the perioperative period. This should include written instructions about how to prepare for the surgery (for example, when to stop anti-platelet or anticoagulant therapies, when to arrive at the hospital). Pictures of an actual surgery, and if possible a video including the sounds of the physiological recordings and procedures, are helpful in preparing the patient for the surgical procedure.

Medical evaluation

The medical evaluation is ordinarily performed by the primary care physician treating the patient. Serious medical conditions, such as unstable cardiac disease, cerebrovascular disease, untreated hypertension, and bleeding disorders, may be contraindications to surgery. The initial evaluation by the movement disorder neurologist should have been received by this physician so that they know what is expected from them and what they can expect for their patient.

Postoperative care

> Patients are given written instructions about postoperative care. Patients are counseled both by the neurosurgeon and the movement disorder neurologist about what to expect after the surgery. Patients are told to stay on their movement disorder medications until seen for initial programming. Specific instructions about how to monitor for postoperative infection are given to the patient and the importance of notifying their physician about any sign of infection is emphasized.

Suture removal is performed 1–2 weeks following surgery, usually by the neurosurgery team.

> Patients should be counseled about the "micro-lesion" effect. Many patients will have transient improvement of their symptoms lasting days to weeks because of this. They should be told about this because as that benefit dissipates, they may become distressed because of the inaccurate presumption that the surgery was unsuccessful.

Initial DBS programming is performed at different postoperative time points at different centers. Some clinicians activate the stimulator within days after surgical implant, though many wait one to several weeks.

Initial programming
Clinical procedures

We generally wait three to four weeks after surgical implant to perform initial programming so that much of the "micro-lesion" effect has resolved. When programming STN DBS patients, patients are told to come into the clinic in the "off" state, not having taken medications since midnight the night before. Again, for patients traveling long distances it may be desirable to stay locally the night before. They should dress comfortably and plan to stay for two to three hours. Descriptions of the methods of initial programming are described in Chapters 6–8. The visit includes a comprehensive history of the postoperative period, including whether the patient experienced even transient improvement of their symptoms, how much "off" time and dyskinesia they are having, and whether they feel there are any adverse effects from the surgery. Examination includes vital signs, a brief neurological examination, motor scales, and an evaluation of dyskinesia. By performing the established scales at each clinical visit, the movement disorder neurologist can reliably assess the clinical state from visit to visit.

> In our center, the movement disorder neurologist does the bulk of the DBS programming, but many centers employ nurses, nurse practitioners, physician assistants, or medical technicians who are trained in DBS programming.

Of course, the movement disorder neurologist is present and available when ancillary personnel are involved. This is both to assess the quality of the programming and also to make medication adjustments.

Since we wait three to four weeks for initial programming when much of the "micro-lesion" effect has resolved, the initial DBS parameters are often adequate to achieve good symptom control until the next scheduled visit in one to three months. For centers performing initial programming earlier, it is possible that patients may need additional programming even earlier.

Education

The patient and care-partners are again cautioned that the first months may be a frustrating time where clinical benefit may not be stable. The appropriate expectations from the surgery are again discussed. It is not unusual, despite the extensive education undertaken during the preoperative period, for patients to inquire about why certain symptoms have not improved. Having the patient view video of their condition prior to the DBS surgery and pointing out the symptoms shown in the video that have improved is helpful in these cases.

The patient is given detailed instructions about what environmental factors may affect their DBS system and what activities or procedures they must avoid (for example, diathermy) and also which medical procedures may be performed. They should have received their patient identification card from the device manufacturer and are instructed to carry this card with them. When traveling through security checkpoints, such as at airports, they may present this card to identify that they have an implantable device that may trigger security alerts. They are assured that the movement disorders neurologist and staff are available to discuss any limitations or precautions that may be needed during medical and dental procedures, and that the manufacturer has a support line available to both patients and medical personnel.

The use of the patient programmer is demonstrated to the patient and care-partners. Patients should attach their name and phone number to it so that if it is lost, it could be returned.

Subsequent programming visits

Clinical procedures

Because of the micro-lesion effect, the patient's clinical condition may not have reached stability for up to three months or even longer. Once the condition of the patient has reached a point of stability, patients will return for visits on a routine basis. If the movement disorder neurologist is the only neurologist for the patient, visits can be at three to six month intervals. If the patient receives care from another neurologist, they may only see the movement disorder neurologist at 6–12 month intervals, mainly to determine if an adjustment of DBS parameters is warranted and to check the battery status and function of the device.

There may be times when patients need to be seen aside from regularly scheduled appointments. This is a challenge for most busy neurology practices, which may be booked for weeks or even months, especially since the visits ordinarily take more time than routine follow-up visits.

> It is wise to reserve some time each week for patients who may need to have additional programming before their regularly scheduled appointment. If this time is not filled with DBS patients, it is usually easy to fill it with other patients a few days before the reserved time.

At follow-up visits, patients undergo a neurological examination, including vital signs, a brief neurological examination, and in many centers the UPDRS (or the appropriate examination for ET and dystonia). Detailed questioning about the presence of "off" time and dyskinesia is done. The effects of medication changes made at prior visits are assessed. When necessary, additional DBS device programming is performed.

Education

Patients will continue to have questions about their device on an on-going basis. With advances in medical treatments using electronic and ultrasonic devices, including some devices used by alternative care practitioners, patients should be told to inquire about any potential effects of these on their DBS systems.

Additional thoughts on management of physician time

The logistical challenge of incorporating a DBS program into a clinical practice is significant. Any neurologist wanting to develop a DBS program must be dedicated and willing to commit the necessary time and energy. Most movement disorder neurologists would agree that caring for patients who have had DBS is more labor intensive than other patients. Because a patient's condition may not be stable for several months, it may be necessary that patients have several DBS programming sessions over the first few months. This may be difficult to arrange in a busy neurology practice. The movement disorder neurologist must prioritize which patients will benefit from additional programming sessions. Many patients with DBS feel that if there is even a slight residual tremor, for example, that they should be able to return the next day for an hour of programming to resolve it. This unrealistic approach is not medically appropriate and will not work in a busy practice. Patients should be counseled that the first few months can be frustrating but that they can be confident that they will reach a point of stability, usually by six months.

On the other hand, patients should be encouraged to call or contact the movement disorder neurologist to discuss their symptoms and any possible side effects from treatment. Often, the situation can be handled on the phone. For example, excessive dyskinesia may be handled by reductions of medication. If a patient has a stimulator that they are able to adjust, patients can be instructed on how to make minor adjustments or to select from a different group of DBS settings in response to changes in their symptoms.

Patient recruitment: establishing a referral base

A program with expert clinicians will only thrive if there is a steady influx of suitable patients to the center. The decision to be evaluated for DBS at a particular clinic is made both by referring neurologists as well as the patients themselves. Therefore, the way to generate referrals to a clinic is to have a program in place to care for DBS patients and to educate physicians and patients in the referral base about DBS. While most potential referring neurologists may assume that the nearest academic program has a clinical DBS program, they may not assume this about a movement disorder neurologist not working at a university program.

The preferred way to establish a referral base is to establish relationships with referring physicians, educating them about the indications and expected outcomes for the treatment. This may include personal one-to-one discussions, as well as presentations at seminars and meetings.

> Perhaps the best way to grow a referral base is to demonstrate to a referring physician that a patient they referred was well cared for at your center.

It is common to have a patient referred for DBS who is not deemed to be a good candidate. In this case, an explanation to the referring neurologist as to the reason for this is necessary. Simply stating that the patient is not a candidate for DBS without adequate explanation will likely result in that neurologist no longer referring patients to the program. On the other hand, if the reasoning behind the decision is clarified, it is likely that the referring neurologist will refer appropriate patients in the future.

The referring neurologist may have concerns about "losing" their patient; in the "real world" this may limit referrals for DBS which, as a result, deny patients appropriate treatment. While, of course, each patient has a right to determine who will manage their care, it should be assumed that patients will continue to be followed by their referring neurologist. These neurologists should understand, however, that during the evaluation period, the movement disorder specialist may need to make medication changes as part of the process of determining if the patient's medical therapy is optimized. In addition, during the initial postoperative period, it is usually necessary for the movement disorder neurologist to adjust medications at DBS programming visits. In a sense, the movement disorder neurologist takes over management of the disease during these periods. Once a stable optimized condition has been achieved, patients may be managed more by their referring neurologist and seen less often by the DBS movement disorder neurologist. This is especially true for patients who travel long distances to the movement disorders center.

Since it is the patient who may also decide to be evaluated at a particular DBS program, physicians involved in DBS programs may volunteer to speak at local patient support groups and symposia. Patients may also be invited to the regularly scheduled informational sessions run by the DBS program.

Conclusions

The decision to embark on a DBS program should be carefully made by neurologists with expertise in movement disorders with the realization that it requires assembling a team of clinicians and that it requires a labor-intensive effort. The clinicians involved will need additional training, so that they can develop an understanding of the details of the selection process and programming techniques. This can be accomplished by reading the literature, attending courses, and by visiting established clinics. It is necessary to develop and abide by an established protocol.

References

1. Hughes AJ, Daniel SE, Kilford L, Lees AJ. Accuracy of clinical diagnosis of idiopathic Parkinson's disease: a clinico-pathological study of 100 cases. *J Neurol Neurosurg Psychiatry* 1992;**55**:181–4.

2. Moro E, Lang AE. Criteria for deep brain stimulation in Parkinson's disease: review and analysis. *Expert Rev Neurother* 2006;**6**(11):1695–1705.

3. Kern DS, Kumar R. Deep brain stimulation. *Neurologist* 2007;**13**(5):237–52.

4. Houeto JL, Damier P, Bejjani PB, et al. Subthalamic stimulation in Parkinson disease: a multidisciplinary approach. *Arch Neurol* 2000;**57**:461–5.

5. Ramig LO, Countryman S, O'Brien C, Hoehn M, Thompson L. Intensive speech treatment for patients with Parkinson's disease: short and long term comparison of two techniques. *Neurology* 1996;**47**:1496–1504.

6. Stankovic I. The effect of physical therapy on balance of patients with Parkinson's disease. *Int J Rehabil Res* 2004;**27**:54–7.

7. Ellis T, De Goede CJ, Feldman RG, et al. Efficacy of a physical therapy program in patients with Parkinson's disease: a randomized controlled trial. *Arch Phys Med Rehabil* 2005;**86**:626–32.

Further reading

Ahlskog JE, Muenter MD. Frequency of levodopa-related dyskinesias and motor fluctuations as estimated from the cumulative literature. *Mov Disord* 2001;**16**(3):448–58.

Bergareche A, De La Puente E, López De Munain A, et al. Prevalence of essential tremor: a door-to-door survey in Bidasoa, Spain. *Neuroepidemiology* 2001;**20**:125–8.

Bower JH, Maraganore DM, McDonnell SK, Rocca WA. Incidence and distribution of parkinsonism in Olmsted County, Minnesota, 1976–1990. *Neurology* 1999;**52**:1214–20.

Cersosimo MG, Koller WC. Essential tremor. In Watts R, Koller W, eds. *Movement Disorders: Neurological Principles and Practice*. New York: McGraw-Hill; 2004:431–57.

Chou KL. Indications for subthalamic nucleus deep brain stimulation surgery. In Baltuch GH, Stern MB, eds. *Deep Brain Stimulation for Parkinson's Disease*. New York: Informa Healthcare USA; 2007:41–54.

Ellis T, De Goede CJ, Feldman RG, et al. Efficacy of a physical therapy program in patients with Parkinson's disease: a randomized controlled trial. *Arch Phys Med Rehabil* 2005;**86**:626–32.

Houeto JL, Damier P, Bejjani PB, et al. Subthalamic stimulation in Parkinson disease: a multidisciplinary approach. *Arch Neurol* 2000;**57**:461–5.

Hughes AJ, Daniel SE, Kilford L, Lees AJ. Accuracy of clinical diagnosis of idiopathic Parkinson's disease: a clinico-pathological study of 100 cases. *J Neurol Neurosurg Psychiatry* 1992;**55**:181–4.

Kern DS, Kumar R. Deep brain stimulation. *Neurologist* 2007;**13**(5):237–52.

Krack P, Batir A, Van Blercom N, et al. Five-year follow-up of bilateral stimulation of the subthalamic nucleus in advanced Parkinson's disease. *N Engl J Med* 2003;**349**(20):1925–34.

Kumar N, Van Gerpen JA, Bower JH, Ahlskog JE. Levodopa-dyskinesia incidence by age of Parkinson's disease onset. *Mov Disord* 2005;**20**(3):342–66.

Louis ED, Barnes L, Albert SM, et al. Correlates of functional disability in essential tremor. *Mov Disord* 2001;**16**(5):914–20.

Mancini ML, Stracci F, Tambasco N, et al. Prevalence of essential tremor in the territory of Lake Trasimeno, Italy: results of a population-based study. *Mov Disord*, 2007;**22**(4):540–5.

Mayeux R, Marder K, Cote LJ, et al. The frequency of idiopathic Parkinson's disease by age, ethnic group, and sex in northern Manhattan, 1988–1993. *Am J Epidemiol* 1995;**142**:820–7.

Müller T, Soitalla D, Russ H, Hock K, Haeger DA. Prevalence and treatment strategies of dyskinesias in patients with Parkinson's disease. *J Neural Transm* 2007;**114**:1023–6.

Pinto S, Gentil M, Krack P, et al. Changes induced by levodopa and subthalamic nucleus stimulation of Parkinsonian speech. *Mov Disord* 2005;**20**(11):1507–15.

Rajput AH, Birdi S. Epidemiology of Parkinson's disease. *Parkinsonism Relat Disord* 1997;**3**(4):175–86.

Rajput AH, Offord KP, Kurland LT. Epidemiologic survey of essential tremor in Rochester. *MN Neurology* 1982;**32**:A128.

Rajput M, Rajput A, Rajput AH. Epidemiology. In Pahwa R, Lyons K, eds. *Handbook of Parkinson's Disease*. New York: Taylor and Francis; 2007:19–27.

Rodriquez-Oroz MC, Obeso JA, Lang AE, et al. Bilateral deep brain stimulation in Parkinson's disease: a multicentre study with 4 years follow-up. *Brain* 2005;**128**:2240–9.

Romito LM, Scerrati M, Contarino MF, et al. Bilateral high frequency subthalamic stimulation in Parkinson's disease: long-term neurological follow-up. *J Neurosurg Sci* 2003;**47**:119–28.

Appendix A: Motor diary

Medication schedule and patient motor fluctuation log

Medication and dose	Time					

Additional instructions:

Please mark an "X" every hour to indicate level of motor function

GRAPH YOUR SYMPTOMS																							
Severe dyskinesia																							
Some dyskinesia																							
Good movement																							
Slow																							
Frozen																							
Indicate when you have taken medication:	6a	7a	8a	9a	10a	11a	12p	1p	2p	3p	4p	5p	6p	7p	8p	9p	10p	11p	12a	1a	2a	3a	4a	5a

Appendix B: Unified Parkinson's Disease Rating Scale

I. Mentation, behavior, and mood

1. **Intellectual impairment**
   0 = None.
   1 = Mild. Consistent forgetfulness with partial recollection of events and no other difficulties.
   2 = Moderate memory loss, with disorientation and moderate difficulty handling complex problems. Mild but definite impairment of function at home with need of occasional prompting.
   3 = Severe memory loss with disorientation for time and often to place. Severe impairment in handling problems.
   4 = Severe memory loss with orientation preserved to person only. Unable to make judgements or solve problems. Requires much help with personal care. Cannot be left alone at all.

2. **Thought disorder (due to dementia or drug intoxication)**
   0 = None.
   1 = Vivid dreaming.
   2 = "Benign" hallucinations with insight retained.
   3 = Occasional to frequent hallucinations or delusions; without insight; could interfere with daily activities.
   4 = Persistent hallucinations, delusions, or florid psychosis. Not able to care for self.

3. **Depression**
   1 = Periods of sadness or guilt greater than normal, never sustained for days or weeks.
   2 = Sustained depression (1 week or more).
   3 = Sustained depression with vegetative symptoms (insomnia, anorexia, weight loss, loss of interest).
   4 = Sustained depression with vegetative symptoms and suicidal thoughts or intent.

4. **Motivation/initiative**
   0 = Normal.
   1 = Less assertive than usual; more passive.
   2 = Loss of initiative or disinterest in elective (nonroutine) activities.
   3 = Loss of initiative or disinterest in day to day (routine) activities.
   4 = Withdrawn, complete loss of motivation.

II. Activities of daily living (for both "on" and "off")

5. **Speech**
   0 = Normal.
   1 = Mildly affected. No difficulty being understood.
   2 = Moderately affected. Sometimes asked to repeat statements.
   3 = Severely affected. Frequently asked to repeat statements.
   4 = Unintelligible most of the time.

6. **Salivation**
   0 = Normal.
   1 = Slight but definite excess of saliva in mouth; may have nighttime drooling.
   2 = Moderately excessive saliva; may have minimal drooling.
   3 = Marked excess of saliva with some drooling.
   4 = Marked drooling, requires constant tissue or handkerchief.

7. **Swallowing**
   0 = Normal.
   1 = Rare choking.
   2 = Occasional choking.

3 = Requires soft food.

4 = Requires NG tube or gastrotomy feeding.

8. **Handwriting**

0 = Normal.

1 = Slightly slow or small.

2 = Moderately slow or small; all words are legible.

3 = Severely affected; not all words are legible.

4 = The majority of words are not legible.

9. **Cutting food and handling utensils**

0 = Normal.

1 = Somewhat slow and clumsy, but no help needed.

2 = Can cut most foods, although clumsy and slow; some help needed.

3 = Food must be cut by someone, but can still feed slowly.

4 = Needs to be fed.

10. **Dressing**

0 = Normal.

1 = Somewhat slow, but no help needed.

2 = Occasional assistance with buttoning, getting arms in sleeves.

3 = Considerable help required, but can do some things alone.

4 = Helpless.

11. **Hygiene**

0 = Normal.

1 = Somewhat slow, but no help needed.

2 = Needs help to shower or bathe; or very slow in hygienic care.

3 = Requires assistance for washing, brushing teeth, combing hair, going to bathroom.

4 = Foley catheter or other mechanical aids.

12. **Turning in bed and adjusting bed clothes**

0 = Normal.

1 = Somewhat slow and clumsy, but no help needed.

2 = Can turn alone or adjust sheets, but with great difficulty.

3 = Can initiate, but not turn or adjust sheets alone.

4 = Helpless.

13. **Falling (unrelated to freezing)**

0 = None.

1 = Rare falling.

2 = Occasionally falls, less than once per day.

3 = Falls an average of once daily.

4 = Falls more than once daily.

14. **Freezing when walking**

0 = None.

1 = Rare freezing when walking; may have start hesitation.

2 = Occasional freezing when walking.

3 = Frequent freezing. Occasionally falls from freezing.

4 = Frequent falls from freezing.

15. **Walking**

0 = Normal.

1 = Mild difficulty. May not swing arms or may tend to drag leg.

2 = Moderate difficulty, but requires little or no assistance.

3 = Severe disturbance of walking, requiring assistance.

4 = Cannot walk at all, even with assistance.

16. **Tremor (symptomatic complaint of tremor in any part of body)**

0 = Absent.

1 = Slight and infrequently present.

2 = Moderate; bothersome to patient.

3 = Severe; interferes with many activities.

4 = Marked; interferes with most activities.

17. **Sensory complaints related to parkinsonism**

0 = None.

1 = Occasionally has numbness, tingling, or mild aching.

2 = Frequently has numbness, tingling, or aching; not distressing.

3 = Frequent painful sensations.

4 = Excruciating pain.

III.   Motor examination

18. **Speech**

0 = Normal.

1 = Slight loss of expression, diction and/or volume.

2 = Monotone, slurred but understandable; moderately impaired.

3 = Marked impairment, difficult to understand.

4 = Unintelligible.

19. **Facial expression**

    0 = Normal.

    1 = Minimal hypomimia, could be normal "Poker Face."

    2 = Slight but definitely abnormal diminution of facial expression.

    3 = Moderate hypomimia; lips parted some of the time.

    4 = Masked or fixed facies with severe or complete loss of facial expression; lips parted 1/4 inch or more.

20. **Tremor at rest (head, upper and lower extremities)**

    0 = Absent.

    1 = Slight and infrequently present.

    2 = Mild in amplitude and persistent. Or moderate in amplitude, but only intermittently present.

    3 = Moderate in amplitude and present most of the time.

    4 = Marked in amplitude and present most of the time.

21. **Action or postural tremor of hands**

    0 = Absent.

    1 = Slight; present with action.

    2 = Moderate in amplitude, present with action.

    3 = Moderate in amplitude with posture holding as well as action.

    4 = Marked in amplitude; interferes with feeding.

22. **Rigidity (Judged on passive movement of major joints with patient relaxed in sitting position. Cogwheeling to be ignored)**

    0 = Absent.

    1 = Slight or detectable only when activated by mirror or other movements.

    2 = Mild to moderate.

    3 = Marked, but full range of motion easily achieved.

    4 = Severe, range of motion achieved with difficulty.

23. **Finger taps (Patient taps thumb with index finger in rapid succession)**

    0 = Normal.

    1 = Mild slowing and/or reduction in amplitude.

    2 = Moderately impaired. Definite and early fatiguing. May have occasional arrests in movement.

    3 = Severely impaired. Frequent hesitation in initiating movements or arrests in ongoing movement.

    4 = Can barely perform the task.

24. **Hand movements (Patient opens and closes hands in rapid succession)**

    0 = Normal.

    1 = Mild slowing and/or reduction in amplitude.

    2 = Moderately impaired. Definite and early fatiguing. May have occasional arrests in movement.

    3 = Severely impaired. Frequent hesitation in initiating movements or arrests in ongoing movement.

    4 = Can barely perform the task.

25. **Rapid alternating movements of hands (Pronation–supination movements of hands, vertically and horizontally, with as large an amplitude as possible, both hands simultaneously)**

    0 = Normal.

    1 = Mild slowing and/or reduction in amplitude.

    2 = Moderately impaired. Definite and early fatiguing. May have occasional arrests in movement.

    3 = Severely impaired. Frequent hesitation in initiating movements or arrests in ongoing movement.

    4 = Can barely perform the task.

26. **Leg agility (Patient taps heel on the ground in rapid succession picking up entire leg. Amplitude should be at least 3 inches)**

    0 = Normal.

    1 = Mild slowing and/or reduction in amplitude.

    2 = Moderately impaired. Definite and early fatiguing. May have occasional arrests in movement.

    3 = Severely impaired. Frequent hesitation in initiating movements or arrests in ongoing movement.

    4 = Can barely perform the task.

27. **Arising from chair (Patient attempts to rise from a straightbacked chair, with arms folded across chest)**
    0 = Normal.
    1 = Slow; or may need more than one attempt.
    2 = Pushes self up from arms of seat.
    3 = Tends to fall back and may have to try more than one time, but can get up without help.
    4 = Unable to arise without help.

28. **Posture**
    0 = Normal erect.
    1 = Not quite erect, slightly stooped posture; could be normal for older person.
    2 = Moderately stooped posture, definitely abnormal; can be slightly leaning to one side.
    3 = Severely stooped posture with kyphosis; can be moderately leaning to one side.
    4 = Marked flexion with extreme abnormality of posture.

29. **Gait**
    0 = Normal.
    1 = Walks slowly, may shuffle with short steps, but no festination (hastening steps) or propulsion.
    2 = Walks with difficulty, but requires little or no assistance; may have some festination, short steps, or propulsion.
    3 = Severe disturbance of gait, requiring assistance.
    4 = Cannot walk at all, even with assistance.

30. **Postural stability (Response to sudden, strong posterior displacement produced by pull on shoulders while patient erect with eyes open and feet slightly apart. Patient is prepared)**
    0 = Normal.
    1 = Retropulsion, but recovers unaided.
    2 = Absence of postural response; would fall if not caught by examiner.
    3 = Very unstable, tends to lose balance spontaneously.
    4 = Unable to stand without assistance.

31. **Body bradykinesia and hypokinesia (Combining slowness, hesitancy, decreased armswing, small amplitude, and poverty of movement in general)**
    0 = None.
    1 = Minimal slowness, giving movement a deliberate character; could be normal for some persons. Possibly reduced amplitude.
    2 = Mild degree of slowness and poverty of movement which is definitely abnormal. Alternatively, some reduced amplitude.
    3 = Moderate slowness, poverty or small amplitude of movement.
    4 = Marked slowness, poverty or small amplitude of movement.

IV. Complications of therapy (in the past week)

A. **Dyskinesias**

32. **Duration: What proportion of the waking day are dyskinesias present? (Historical information)**
    0 = None
    1 = 1–25% of day
    2 = 26–50% of day
    3 = 51–75% of day
    4 = 76–100% of day

33. **Disability: How disabling are the dyskinesias? (Historical information; may be modified by office examination)**
    0 = Not disabling
    1 = Mildly disabling
    2 = Moderately disabling
    3 = Severely disabling
    4 = Completely disabled

34. **Painful dyskinesias: How painful are the dyskinesias?**
    0 = No painful dyskinesias
    1 = Slight
    2 = Moderate
    3 = Severe
    4 = Marked

35. **Presence of early morning dystonia (Historical information)**
    0 = No
    1 = Yes

B. **Clinical fluctuations**

36. **Are "off" periods predictable?**
    0 = No
    1 = Yes

37. **Are "off" periods unpredictable?**
    0 = No
    1 = Yes

38. **Do "off" periods come on suddenly, within a few seconds?**
    0 = No
    1 = Yes

39. **What proportion of the waking day is the patient "off" on average?**
    0 = None
    1 = 1–25% of day
    2 = 26–50% of day
    3 = 51–75% of day
    4 = 76–100% of day

C. **Other complications**

40. **Does the patient have anorexia, nausea, or vomiting?**
    0 = No
    1 = Yes

41. **Any sleep disturbances, such as insomnia or hypersomnolence?**
    0 = No
    1 = Yes

42. **Does the patient have symptomatic orthostasis? (Record the patient's blood pressure, height and weight on the scoring form)**
    0 = No
    1 = Yes

V. Modified Hoehn and Yahr staging

Stage 0 = No signs of disease.
Stage 1 = Unilateral disease.
Stage 1.5 = Unilateral plus axial involvement.
Stage 2 = Bilateral disease, without impairment of balance.
Stage 2.5 = Mild bilateral disease, with recovery on pull test.
Stage 3 = Mild to moderate bilateral disease; some postural instability; physically independent.
Stage 4 = Severe disability; still able to walk or stand unassisted.
Stage 5 = Wheelchair bound or bedridden unless aided.

VI. Schwab and England Activities of Daily Living Scale

100% = Completely independent. Able to do all chores without slowness, difficulty, or impairment. Essentially normal. Unaware of any difficulty.
90% = Completely independent. Able to do all chores with some degree of slowness, difficulty, and impairment. Might take twice as long. Beginning to be aware of difficulty.
80% = Completely independent in most chores. Takes twice as long. Conscious of difficulty and slowness.
70% = Not completely independent. More difficulty with some chores. Three to four times as long in some. Must spend a large part of the day with chores.
60% = Some dependency. Can do most chores, but exceedingly slowly and with much effort. Errors; some impossible.
50% = More dependent. Help with half, slower, etc. Difficulty with everything.
40% = Very dependent. Can assist with all chores, but few alone.
30% = With effort, now and then does a few chores alone or begins alone. Much help needed.
20% = Nothing alone. Can be a slight help with some chores. Severe invalid.
10% = Totally dependent, helpless. Complete invalid.
0% = Vegetative functions such as swallowing, bladder and bowel functions are not functioning. Bedridden.

Source: Reproduced with permission from WE MOVE at www.mdvu.org and Professor Stanley Fahn, reproduced from Fahn S, Elton RL, Members of the UPDRS Development Committee. The Unified Parkinson's Disease Rating Scale. In Fahn S, Marsden CD, Calne DB, Goldstein M, eds: *Recent Developments in Parkinson's Disease, Vol. 2.* Florham Park, NJ: Macmillan Healthcare Information, 1987. pp. 153–163, 293–304.

Appendix C: Abnormal Involuntary Movement Scale

Patient's Name (Please print) _____   **Patient's ID information** _____

	None, normal	Minimal (may be extreme normal)	Mild	Moderate	Severe
Facial and Oral Movements					
1. Muscles of Facial Expression e.g., movements of forehead, eyebrows, periorbital area, cheeks; include frowning, blinking, smiling, grimacing	☐ 0	☐ 1	☐ 2	☐ 3	☐ 4
2. Lips and Perioral Area e.g., puckering, pouting, smacking	☐ 0	☐ 1	☐ 2	☐ 3	☐ 4
3. Jaw e.g., biting, clenching, chewing, mouth opening, lateral movement	☐ 0	☐ 1	☐ 2	☐ 3	☐ 4
4. Tongue Rate only increases in movement both in and out of mouth NOT inability to sustain movement	☐ 0	☐ 1	☐ 2	☐ 3	☐ 4
Extremity Movements					
5. Upper (arms, wrists, hands, fingers) Include choreic movements (i.e., rapid, objectively purposeless, irregular, spontaneous); athetoid movements (i.e., slow, irregular, complex, serpentine) DO NOT include tremor (i.e., repetitive, regular, rhythmic)	☐ 0	☐ 1	☐ 2	☐ 3	☐ 4
6. Lower (legs, knees, ankles, toes) e.g., lateral knee movement, foot tapping, heel dropping, foot squirming, inversion and eversion of foot	☐ 0	☐ 1	☐ 2	☐ 3	☐ 4
Trunk Movements					
7. Neck, shoulders, hips e.g., rocking, twisting, squirming, pelvic gyrations	☐ 0	☐ 1	☐ 2	☐ 3	☐ 4

SCORING:

- Score the highest amplitude or frequency in a movement on the 0–4 scale, not the average

- Score Activated Movements the same way; do not lower those numbers as was proposed at one time

- A POSITIVE AIMS EXAMINATION IS A SCORE OF 2 IN TWO OR MORE MOVEMENTS or a SCORE OF 3 OR 4 IN A SINGLE MOVEMENT

- Do not sum the scores: e.g., a patient who scores 1 in four movements DOES NOT have a positive AIMS score of 4

Overall Severity

		0	1	2	3	4
8.	Severity of abnormal movements	☐	☐	☐	☐	☐
9.	Incapacitation due to abnormal movements	☐	☐	☐	☐	☐
		No awareness	Aware, no distress	Aware, mild distress	Aware, moderate distress	Aware, severe distress
10.	Patient's awareness of abnormal movements (rate only patient's report)	☐	☐	☐	☐	☐

Dental Status

		Yes	No
11.	Current problems with teeth and/or dentures?	☐	☐
12.	Does patient usually wear dentures?	☐	☐

Source: Reproduced from Guy W: *ECDEN Assessment Manual for Psychopharmacology – Revised* (DHEW publ No ADM 76-338), US Department of Health, Education, and Welfare; 1976. (See: http://flmedicaidbh.fmhi.usf.edu/pdf/AIMS_Quest.pdf)

Appendix D: PDQ-39 questionnaire

Please check *one box* for each question

Due to having Parkinson's disease, how often <u>during the last month</u> have you. . . .	Never	Occasionally	Sometimes	Often	Always or cannot do at all
1 Had difficulty doing the leisure activities you would like to do?	☐	☐	☐	☐	☐
2 Had difficulty looking after your home, for example, housework, cooking or yardwork?	☐	☐	☐	☐	☐
3 Had difficulty carrying grocery bags?	☐	☐	☐	☐	☐
4 Had problems walking half a mile?	☐	☐	☐	☐	☐
5 Had problems walking 100 yards (approximately 1 block)?	☐	☐	☐	☐	☐
6 Had problems getting around the house as easily as you would like?	☐	☐	☐	☐	☐
7 Had difficulty getting around in public places?	☐	☐	☐	☐	☐
8 Needed someone else to accompany you when you went out?	☐	☐	☐	☐	☐
9 Felt frightened or worried about falling over in public?	☐	☐	☐	☐	☐
10 Been confined to the house more than you would like?	☐	☐	☐	☐	☐
11 Had difficulty showering and bathing?	☐	☐	☐	☐	☐
12 Had difficulty dressing?	☐	☐	☐	☐	☐
13 Had difficulty with buttons or shoelaces?	☐	☐	☐	☐	☐
14 Had problems writing clearly?	☐	☐	☐	☐	☐
15 Had difficulty cutting up your food?	☐	☐	☐	☐	☐
16 Had difficulty holding a drink without spilling it?	☐	☐	☐	☐	☐
17 Felt depressed?	☐	☐	☐	☐	☐
18 Felt isolated and lonely?	☐	☐	☐	☐	☐
19 Felt weepy or tearful?	☐	☐	☐	☐	☐
20 Felt angry or bitter?	☐	☐	☐	☐	☐

Please check that you have checked <u>one box for each question</u> before going on to the next page

Please check *one box* for each question

Due to having Parkinson's disease, how often <u>during the last month</u> have you. . . .	Never	Occasionally	Sometimes	Often	Always or cannot do at all
21 Felt anxious?	☐	☐	☐	☐	☐
22 Felt worried about your future?	☐	☐	☐	☐	☐
23 Felt you had to hide your Parkinson's from people?	☐	☐	☐	☐	☐
24 Avoided situations which involve eating or drinking in public?	☐	☐	☐	☐	☐
25 Felt embarrassed in public?	☐	☐	☐	☐	☐
26 Felt worried by other people's reaction to you?	☐	☐	☐	☐	☐
27 Had problems with your close personal relationships?	☐	☐	☐	☐	☐
28 Lacked the support you needed from your spouse or partner?	☐	☐	☐	☐	☐
If you do not have a spouse or partner, please check here			☐		
29 Lacked the support you needed from your family or close friends?	☐	☐	☐	☐	☐
30 Unexpectedly fallen asleep during the day?	☐	☐	☐	☐	☐
31 Had problems with your concentration, for example when reading or watching TV?	☐	☐	☐	☐	☐
32 Felt your memory was failing?	☐	☐	☐	☐	☐
33 Had distressing dreams or hallucinations?	☐	☐	☐	☐	☐
34 Had difficulty speaking?	☐	☐	☐	☐	☐
35 Felt unable to communicate effectively?	☐	☐	☐	☐	☐
36 Felt ignored by people?	☐	☐	☐	☐	☐
37 Had painful muscle cramps or spasms?	☐	☐	☐	☐	☐
38 Had aches and pains in your joints or body?	☐	☐	☐	☐	☐
39 Felt uncomfortably hot or cold?	☐	☐	☐	☐	☐

Please check that you have checked <u>one box for each question</u>

Appendix E: Montreal Cognitive Assessment Test – English

MONTREAL COGNITIVE ASSESSMENT (MOCA)

NAME :
Education :
Sex :
Date of birth :
DATE :

VISUOSPATIAL / EXECUTIVE				POINTS

Copy cube

Draw CLOCK (Ten past eleven) (3 points)

[ ]   [ ]   [ ]   [ ]   [ ]   /5
Contour Numbers Hands

NAMING

[ ]   [ ]   [ ]   /3

MEMORY Read list of words, subject must repeat them. Do 2 trials, even if 1st trial is successful. Do a recall after 5 minutes.		FACE	VELVET	CHURCH	DAISY	RED	No points
	1st trial						
	2nd trial						

ATTENTION Read list of digits (1 digit/ sec).	Subject has to repeat them in the forward order	[ ] 2 1 8 5 4	/2
	Subject has to repeat them in the backward order	[ ] 7 4 2	

Read list of letters. The subject must tap with his hand at each letter A. No points if ≥ 2 errors
[ ] F B A C M N A A J K L B A F A K D E A A A J A M O F A A B   /1

Serial 7 subtraction starting at 100	[ ] 93	[ ] 86	[ ] 79	[ ] 72	[ ] 65	/3
	4 or 5 correct subtractions: **3 pts**, 2 or 3 correct: **2 pts**, 1 correct: **1 pt**, 0 correct: **0 pt**					

LANGUAGE	Repeat : I only know that John is the one to help today. [ ] The cat always hid under the couch when dogs were in the room. [ ]	/2
	Fluency / Name maximum number of words in one minute that begin with the letter F [ ] _____ (N ≥ 11 words)	/1

ABSTRACTION	Similarity between e.g. banana - orange = fruit [ ] train – bicycle [ ] watch - ruler	/2

DELAYED RECALL	Has to recall words WITH NO CUE	FACE [ ]	VELVET [ ]	CHURCH [ ]	DAISY [ ]	RED [ ]	Points for UNCUED recall only	/5
Optional	Category cue							
	Multiple choice cue							

ORIENTATION	[ ] Date	[ ] Month	[ ] Year	[ ] Day	[ ] Place	[ ] City	/6

© Z.Nasreddine MD   Version 7.1   www.mocatest.org   Normal ≥26 / 30   TOTAL _____/30

Add 1 point if ≤12 yr edu

Administered by: _____

Appendix F: Geriatric Depression Scale

Mood scale (short form)

Choose the best answer for how you have felt over the past week:

1. Are you basically satisfied with your life? YES / **NO**
2. Have you dropped many of your activities and interests? **YES** / NO
3. Do you feel that your life is empty? **YES** / NO
4. Do you often get bored? **YES** / NO
5. Are you in good spirits most of the time? YES / **NO**
6. Are you afraid that something bad is going to happen to you? **YES** / NO
7. Do you feel happy most of the time? YES / **NO**
8. Do you often feel helpless? **YES** / NO
9. Do you prefer to stay at home, rather than going out and doing new things? **YES** / NO
10. Do you feel you have more problems with memory than most? **YES** / NO
11. Do you think it is wonderful to be alive now? YES / **NO**
12. Do you feel pretty worthless the way you are now? **YES** / NO
13. Do you feel full of energy? YES / **NO**
14. Do you feel that your situation is hopeless? **YES** / NO
15. Do you think that most people are better off than you are? **YES** / NO

Answers in **bold** indicate depression. Although differing sensitivities and specificities have been obtained across studies, for clinical purposes a score >5 points is suggestive of depression and should warrant a follow-up interview. Scores >10 are almost always depression.

Source: Reproduced with permission from the Stanford/VA/NIA Aging Clinical Research Center (ACRC) website (see: http://www.stanford.edu/~yesavage/GDS.html)

Appendix G: Burke–Fahn–Marsden Dystonia Rating Scale

Region	Provoking factor		Severity	Weight factor	Product	
Eyes	0–4	x		0–4	0.5	0–8
Mouth	0–4	x		0–4	0.5	0–8
Speech						
Swallow	0–4	x		0–4	1.0	0–16
Neck	0–4	x		0–4	0.5	0–8
R arm	0–4	x		0–4	1.0	0–16
L arm	0–4	x		0–4	1.0	0–16
Trunk	0–4	x		0–4	1.0	0–16
R leg	0–4	x		0–4	1.0	0–16
L leg	0–4	x		0–4	1.0	0–16

Sum:

Maximum=120

I. **Provoking Factor**
A. **General**
0. No dystonia at rest or with action
1. Dystonia only with particular action
2. Dystonia with many actions
3. Dystonia on action of distant part of body or intermittently at rest
4. Dystonia present at rest

B. **Speech and swallowing**
0. Occasional, either or both
1. Frequent either
2. Frequent one and occasional other
3. Frequent both

II. **Severity Factors Eyes**
0. No dystonia
1. Slight. Occasional blinking
2. Mild. Frequent blinking without prolonged spasms of eye closure
3. Moderate. Prolonged spasms of eyelid closure, but eyes open most of the time
4. Severe. Prolonged spasms of eyelid closure, with eyes closed at least 30% of the time

Mouth
0. No dystonia present
1. Slight. Occasional grimacing or other mouth movements (e.g., jaw opened or clenched; tongue movement)
2. Mild. Movement present less than 50% of the time

Speech and swallowing
0. Normal
1. Slightly involved; speech easily understood or occasional choking
2. Some difficulty in understanding speech or frequent choking
3. Marked difficulty in understanding speech or inability to swallow firm foods
4. Complete or almost complete anarthria, or marked difficulty swallowing soft foods and liquids

Neck
0. No dystonia present
1. Slight. Occasional pulling
2. Obvious torticollis, but mild
3. Moderate pulling
4. Extreme pulling

Arm
0. No dystonia present
1. Slight dystonia. Clinically insignificant
2. Mild. Obvious dystonia, but not disabling
3. Moderate. Able to grasp, with some manual function
4. Severe. No useful grasp

Trunk
0. No dystonia present
1. Slight bending; clinically insignificant
2. Definite bending, but not interfering with standing or walking
3. Moderate bending; interfering with standing or walking
4. Extreme bending of trunk preventing standing or walking

Leg
0. No dystonia present
1. Slight dystonia, but not causing impairment; clinically insignificant
2. Mild dystonia. Walks briskly and unaided
3. Moderate dystonia. Severely impairs walking or requires assistance
4. Severe. Unable to stand or walk on involved leg

Source: Reproduced with permission from WE MOVE © WE MOVE 2005. (See: http://www.mdvu.org/library/ratingscales/)

Appendix H: Toronto Western Spasmodic Torticollis Rating Scale

I. Torticollis Severity Scale

A. **Maximal Excursion**
1. **Rotation** (*turn: right or left*)
   - 0 = None [0°]
   - 1 = Slight [¼–¼ range, 1°–22°]
   - 2 = Mild [¼–½ range, 23°–45°]
   - 3 = Moderate [½–¾ range, 46°–67°]
   - 4 = Severe [>¾ range, 68°–90°]
2. **Laterocollis** (*tilt: right or left, exclude shoulder elevation*)
   - 0 = None [0°]
   - 1 = Mild [1°–15°]
   - 2 = Moderate [16°–35°]
   - 3 = Severe [> 35°]
3. **Anterocollis/Retrocollis** (*a or b*)
   a. **Anterocollis**
   - 0 = None
   - 1 = Mild downward deviation of chin
   - 2 = Moderate downward deviation (approximates ½ possible range)
   - 3 = Severe (chin approximates chest)
   b. **Retrocollis**
   - 0 = None
   - 1 = Mild backward deviation of vertex with upward deviation of chin
   - 2 = Moderate backward deviation (approximates ½ possible range)
   - 3 = Severe (approximates full range)
4. **Lateral shift** (*right or left*)
   - 0 = Absent
   - 1 = Present
5. **Sagittal shift** (*forward or backward*)
   - 0 = Absent
   - 1 = Present

B. **Duration Factor** (*Weighted × 2*)
   - 0 = None
   - 1 = Occasional deviation (< 25% of the time, most often submaximal)
   - 2 = Occasional deviation (< 25% of the time, often maximal) **or** Intermittent deviation (25%–50% of the time, most often submaximal)
   - 3 = Intermittent deviation (25%–50% of the time, often maximal) **or** Frequent deviation (50%–75% of the time, most often submaximal)
   - 4 = Frequent deviation (50%–75% of the time, often maximal) **or** Constant deviation (>75% of the time, most often submaximal)
   - 5 = Constant deviation (>75% of the time, often maximal)
C. **Effect of Sensory Tricks**
   - 0 = Complete relief by one or more tricks
   - 1 = Partial or only limited relief by tricks
   - 2 = Little or no benefit from tricks
D. **Shoulder Elevation/Anterior Displacement**
   - 0 = Absent
   - 1 = Mild (< ⅓ possible range, intermittent or constant)
   - 2 = Moderate (⅓–⅔ possible range and constant, > 75% of the time) **or** Severe (> ⅔ possible range and intermittent)
   - 3 = Severe and constant
E. **Range of Motion** (*without aid of sensory tricks*)
   - 0 = Able to move to extreme opposite position
   - 1 = Able to move head well past midline but not to extreme opposite position
   - 2 = Able to move head barely past midline

3 — Able to move head toward but not past midline

4 = Barely able to move head beyond abnormal posture

F. **Time** *(up to 60 seconds) for which patient is able to maintain head within 10° of neutral position without using sensory tricks (mean of two attempts)*

0 = > 60 seconds

1 = 46–60 seconds

2 = 31–45 seconds

3 = 16–30 seconds

4 = < 15 seconds

II. Disability Scale (maximum = 20)

A. **Work** *(occupation or housework/home management)*

0 = No difficulty

1 = Normal work expectations with satisfactory performance at usual level of occupation but some interference by torticollis

2 = Most activities unlimited, selected activities very difficult and hampered but still possible with satisfactory performance

3 = Working at lower than usual occupation level; most activities hampered, all possible but with less than satisfactory performance in some activities

4 = Unable to engage in voluntary or gainful employment; still able to perform some domestic responsibilities satisfactorily

5 = Marginal or no ability to perform domestic responsibilities

B. **Activities of Daily Living** *(e.g., feeding, dressing, or hygiene, including washing, shaving, makeup, etc.)*

0 = No difficulty with any activity

1 = Activities unlimited but some interference by torticollis

2 = Most activities unlimited, selected activities very difficult and hampered but still possible using simple tricks

3 = Most activities hampered or laborious but still possible; may use extreme tricks

4 = All activities impaired; some impossible or require assistance

5 = Dependent on others in most self-care tasks

C. **Driving**

0 = No difficulty (or has never driven a car)

1 = Unlimited ability to drive but bothered by torticollis

2 = Unlimited ability to drive but requires tricks (including touching or holding face, holding head against head rest) to control torticollis

3 = Can drive only short distances

4 = Usually cannot drive because of torticollis

5 = Unable to drive and cannot ride in a car for long stretches as a passenger because of torticollis

D. **Reading**

1 = Unlimited ability to read in normal seated position but bothered by torticollis

2 = Unlimited ability to read in normal seated position but requires use of tricks to control torticollis

3 = Unlimited ability to read but requires extensive measures to control torticollis **or** is able to read only in nonseated position (e.g., lying down)

4 = Limited ability to read because of torticollis despite tricks

5 = Unable to read more than a few sentences because of torticollis

E. **Television**

0 = No difficulty

1 = Unlimited ability to watch television in normal seated position but bothered by torticollis

2 = Unlimited ability to watch television in normal seated position but requires use of tricks to control torticollis

3 = Unlimited ability to watch television but requires extensive measures to control torticollis **or** is able to view only in nonseated position (e.g., lying down)

4 = Limited ability to watch television because of torticollis

5 = Unable to watch television more than a few minutes because of torticollis

F. **Activities Outside the Home** *(e.g., shopping, walking about, movies, dining, and other recreational activities)*

0 = No difficulty

1 = Unlimited activities but bothered by torticollis

2 = Unlimited activities but requires simple tricks to accomplish

3 = Accomplishes activities only when accompanied by others because of torticollis

4 = Limited activities outside the home: certain activities impossible or given up because of torticollis

5 = Rarely if, ever engages in activities outside the home

III. Pain Scale (maximum = 20)

A. **Severity of Pain** Rate the severity of neck due to ST during the last week on a scale of 0–10 where a score of 0 represents no pain and 10 represents the most excruciating pain imaginable. Score calculated as: (worst + best + (2*usual))/4

Best_____

Worst_____

Usual_____

B. **Duration of Pain**

    0 = None

    1 = Present < 10% of the time

    2 = Present 10%–25% of the time

    3 = Present 26%–50% of the time

    4 = Present 51%–75% of the time

    5 = Present > 76% of the time

C. **Disability Due to Pain**

    0 = No limitation or interference from pain

1 = Pain is quite bothersome but not a source of disability

2 = Pain definitely interferes with some tasks but is not a major contributor to disability

3 = Pain accounts for some (less than half) but not all of disability

4 = Pain is a major source of difficulty with activities; separate from this, head pulling is also a source of some (less than half) disability

5 = Pain is the major source of disability, without it most impaired activities could be performed quite satisfactorily despite the head pulling

1.   Consly ES, Lang AE. Clinical assessments of patients with cervical dystonia. In: Jankovic J, Halleti M, eds. *Therapy with Botulinum Toxin*. New York, NY: Marcel Dekker, Inc.; 1994: 211–37.

Source: Reproduced with permission from WE MOVE © WE MOVE. (See: http://www.wemove.org)

Appendix I: GPi DBS programming data sheet

PATIENT: _____ DATE: _____

SIDE: **L R** Surgery date: _____ Date of last parameter change: _____

Present settings: _____ electrodes; _____ V/mA; _____ μs; _____ Hz

Impedance (Ω)	Current (μA/mA)	Electrode	Amplitude threshold for corticospinal or corticobulbar tract activation	Threshold for phosphenes	Other amplitude thresholds for beneficial and adverse effects
		Monopolar 0			
		Monopolar 1			
		Monopolar 2			
		Monopolar 3			
		Other			
		Other			
		Other			

Medications:

Final stimulation parameters at end of this session: _____ electrodes; _____ V/mA; _____ μs; _____ Hz

Beneficial effects:

Adverse effects:

Comments:

Appendix J: STN DBS programming data sheet

PATIENT: _____ DATE: _____

SIDE: **L R** Surgery date: _____ Date of last parameter change: _____

Present settings: _____ electrodes; _____ V/mA; _____ µs; _____ Hz

Impedance (Ω)	Current (µA/mA)	Electrode	Amplitude threshold for transient paresthesia	Amplitude threshold for persistent (>1 min.) paresthesia	Amplitude threshold for corticospinal or corticobulbar tract activation	Other amplitude thresholds for beneficial and adverse effects
		Monopolar 0				
		Monopolar 1				
		Monopolar 2				
		Monopolar 3				
		Other				
		Other				
		Other				

Medications:

Final stimulation parameters at end of this session: _____ electrodes; _____ V/mA; _____ µs; _____ Hz

Beneficial effects:

Adverse effects:

Comments:

Appendix K: Vim DBS programming data sheet

PATIENT: _____ DATE: _____

SIDE: **L R** Surgery date: _____ Date of last parameter change: _____

Present settings: _____ electrodes; _____ V/mA; _____ µs; _____ Hz

Impedance (Ω)	Current (µA/mA)	Electrode	Amplitude threshold for transient paresthesia	Amplitude threshold for persistent (>1 min.) paresthesia	Amplitude thresholds for start of tremor relief/best tremor relief and degree of tremor control	Other amplitude thresholds for beneficial and adverse effects
		Monopolar 0				
		Monopolar 1				
		Monopolar 2				
		Monopolar 3				
		Other				
		Other				
		Other				

Medications:

Final stimulation parameters at end of this session: _____ electrodes; _____ V/mA; _____ µs; _____ Hz

Beneficial effects:

Adverse effects:

Comments:

Appendix L: DBS programming tracking form

Patient Name:

Diagnosis:
Target:

L/R

Date	Electrodes				Amp	PW	R	Comments
	Case	0	1	2	3			

L/R

Electrodes					Amp	PW	R	Comments
Case	4	5	6	7				

Appendix M: Tremor Rating Scale

Tremor Assessment Form

Patient name: _____   Date: _____

Dominant hand (circle one):   R   L   Physician: _____

Description of Tremor

Location	Severity	When present?			
Face/Chin		R	P	K	
Voice		R	P	K	
Tongue		R	P	K	
Head/Neck		R	P	K	
Trunk		R	P	K	T
Right arm		R	P	K	T
Left arm		R	P	K	T
Right leg		R	P	K	T
Left leg		R	P	K	T

Severity:
0 – none   R = resting
1 – mild   P = postural
2 – moderate   K = kinetic
3 – severe   T = task-specific
4 – incapacitating

Current Medications for Tremor

Medications	Dose	Frequency

Patient's Response to Therapy

_____

_____

_____

Patient's Level of Difficulty with:

_____working   _____speaking   _____writing

_____dressing   _____fine movements   _____depression due to tremor

_____pouring   _____hygiene   _____anxiety due to tremor

_____eating   _____drinking   _____embarrassment

_____involvement in social functions

Archimedes Spiral

Left hand Physician rating _____   Right hand Physician rating _____

Severity:
0-none
1-mild
2-moderate
3-severe
4-incapacitating

Line Drawing

R •

L •

•

•

Left hand Physician rating _____   Right hand Physician rating _____

Handwriting Sample

_____

Speech and Voice Exam

Conversational speech   Physician rating _____

Count to 10   Physician rating _____

Sustained "eeeee" for 5 seconds   Physician rating_____

Source: Reproduced with permission from WE MOVE © WE MOVE.
(See: http://www.mdvu.org/library/ratingscales/)

Index